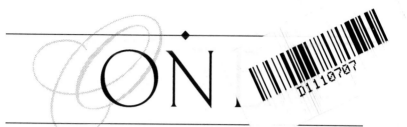

ON A
TATTERED
ANGEL

*A touching true story
of the power of love*

BLAINE M. YORGASON

Shadow Mountain
Salt Lake City, Utah

Recipient of the American Family Institute Literary Award for Nonfiction: "Presented to a work of nonfiction that contributes to the body of literature promoting families as the central units of society and that espouses the enduring values of virtuous living."

© 1995, 1998 Blaine M. Yorgason

Visit us at shadowmountain.com

First published in hardbound (revised edition) 1998
First published in paperbound (revised edition) 2003

Library of Congress Cataloging-in-Publication Data
  Yorgason, Blaine M., 1942-
     One tattered angel : a touching true story of the power of love /
  Blaine M. Yorgason.
          p.   cm.
     "Revised and enlarged."
     ISBN 1-57345-392-7 (hbk.)
     ISBN 1-59038-096-7 (pbk.)
     1. Yorgason, Charity Afton, 1988-   —Health.   2. Hydrocephalus in
  infants—Patients—Utah—Salt Lake City—Biography.
  I. Title.
  RJ496.H9Y678   1998
  362.1'9892858843'0092—dc21
     [b]   98-8352
                                                                       CIP

Printed in the United States of America   3170
Alexander's Printing, Salt Lake City, UT

10   9   8

For Charity and my beloved Kathy,
two of heaven's daughters.
For all the Christlike men and women
who have given Charity and us their love
through service.
And for all tattered angels everywhere.

Musings after First Meeting Charity

Beautiful Sunshine
His image, her countenance
An angel baby
Charity

—David Bestenlehner, Charity's brother-in-law

CONTENTS

Introduction

I have thought about this book for a long time: ten years, to be exact. For most of that time I never expected to write the whole thing. It seemed too close, too personal. That I am now doing so amazes me. It also amazes me that the idea of *not* writing it suddenly seems selfish and maybe even unkind.

Why? Because I have been forever blessed by a tiny but incredible slice of eternity that God has given me—an experience that I can no longer, in good conscience, hold to myself.

Some names and scenes will be changed and dialogue reconstructed, but what follows will be as true an account as I am able to make. Almost in fear and trembling, therefore, yet with hopeful anticipation, I present Charity's story.

An Unusual Warning

"Honey," Kathy whispered urgently, "are you awake?"

"Mmmph," I replied groggily as I rolled over. "I . . . am now."

"I just had the most wonderful dream! Wake up so I can tell you about it."

It was the fall of 1983, so early that the light was barely showing outside our window, and I was not in a joyful mood. In fact, I remember dampening Kathy's excitement a little by telling her that anything dreamed that early in the morning sounded more like a nightmare. She remained convinced, however, that the dream was significant. And she wanted me to know of it.

I should state here a fact that has become more and more clear to me through the years: I am one of those fortunate few who somehow managed, through either remarkable luck or the direct intervention of heaven, to entice a woman of vast spiritual superiority to spend her life with me. Where I believe in righteousness and steadfastness and courage, she embodies them. Where I give lip service to the principles of love and compassion, she reaches out to others in a way I cannot even begin to comprehend. And when I bring suffering upon myself or others because of my own foolishness, she is always there, lifting me, forgiving me, loving me.

"All right," I finally grumbled, leaning on my elbow and trying to focus my eyes in the early-morning gloom, "tell me your nightmare."

"It was a wonderful dream," she began, staring up at the ceiling with a soft smile on her face. "I dreamed we were going to have another baby—a little girl."

"Yep," I breathed, collapsing back onto my pillow with an exaggerated sigh. "Sounds like a nightmare, all right."

"Blaine!"

Recovering from Kathy's light blow, I grinned. "I'm sorry, hon. I'll be serious."

"Yeah, right, you will."

"I mean it. I'll try. Now, let's hear about this little girl we're supposed to have that we both know we can't have."

I was only partly teasing, for indeed we both knew Kathy could never give birth to another child. A ruptured uterus during labor and an emergency hysterectomy following the birth of our sixth child, Michelle, had rendered her physically incapable. Yet here she was, eight years later, all excited about another baby. "Baby hungry" was a term she often used when holding other women's children, and that was obviously her problem now. About all I could do, therefore, was smile and listen and wait for her "hunger" to pass.

Gazing at my sweetheart in the dim light of dawn, I could see the hint of gray in her hair, the wrinkles beginning to appear on her face, and the sagging signs of exhaustion both in and beneath her lovely eyes (no doubt due to the trauma of rearing one stubborn husband and a stampeding horde of teenage and sub-teenage children). Had it really been nineteen years, I wondered, since I had first seen her coming through the doorway of that store and known, instantly and with absolute certainty, that she and I were supposed to be one? It seemed such a short time ago that, frightened beyond belief, I had approached her with my hand outstretched, introduced myself, and asked her for a date.

Demonstrating what some would consider great wisdom, she had turned me down flat. Knowing what I "knew" of our future, however, kept me going, and two weeks later we were engaged. Six weeks after that we were married. ("Don't you ever do this!" I have warned our children since. "After all, it took us two years just to get our names straight!") And for nineteen years we had together enjoyed the happiness and weathered the vicissitudes of life. Mostly, though, we had been happy. Our six children, though a handful, were maturing (more or less) into wonderful young adults, and I sort of expected that Kathy and I were about ready for some years of peace and freedom.

But now she had been given this troublesome dream.

"She was a newly born baby, honey, very tiny and so cute. I had her in an infant seat, but she had on no clothing but a diaper and a thin receiving blanket, and I was worried about her getting cold. Though she looked perfectly normal and healthy, I was trying desperately to get her to a hospital for care. But for some reason I kept falling down, getting the baby all wet and cold. Yet she never cried or complained. She just smiled and loved me.

"Another thing was that people kept stopping me to see her and tell me how beautiful she was. And she was beautiful, Blaine! She had dark hair, dark eyes, a beautiful complexion, and an incredible smile—she was so perfect, and I was so proud of her. But I had to get her to that hospital—"

"Why?" I asked, trying not to sound too interested.

"I don't know. She looked perfect, but she seemed to have a health problem I couldn't see."

"Sounds like a strange dream, Kath. Like I said, a nightmare, something we don't want anything to do with."

"You didn't feel that way in the dream."

"There's more?" I groaned, realizing she hadn't yet mentioned any part I had played in her dream.

Kathy smiled at my hammed-up distress. "A little. When I finally got to the hospital, you were there waiting for me. You took our little girl from me, hon, and told me that everything was going to be just fine. You absolutely loved her! I have never seen such a look of pure happiness on your face as when you held her."

"I doubt that," I said, once again dropping back onto the bed.

"Why?"

"Because I hate hospitals! I don't like even being around sick people. You can bet I wouldn't be happy there."

"It wasn't the hospital that made you happy, silly. It was our little daughter. You loved her more than I can say, and that love glowed all over you just like a light."

"I doubt that, too," I declared, feeling a little less jovial. "Think about it, Kath. For us to get a little girl means we would have to adopt her. Occasionally I've thought about adoption, and, to tell you the truth, I don't think I could love someone else's child the way I love my own."

"Sure you could."

"No I couldn't," I declared, warming to the subject. "But there's another problem, a much larger one. We've already had our family. They're all growing up now, finally giving us the freedom to go off by ourselves, without worry, to enjoy life. Besides, my books are doing well, very well. Doubleday has accepted *Massacre at Salt Creek* for publication, and the stage play based on *Charlie's Monument* is touring the western United States. The movie based on *The Windwalker* has done great, too, and now that it has won those awards we might even see more of my books made into movies. I think we need to take advantage of every opportunity we have to keep going."

I did, too. I had ended my high-school teaching career six years before and had moved my family to Utah, a state overflowing with gorgeous mountains and deserts. Here, I felt, not only could I pursue my studies of western American history but, inspired by the scenic grandeur around me, I could begin writing the historical novels that were agitating my mind. During our six years in Utah my writing career had gone better than I had hoped, much better, and I could see no reason it shouldn't continue.

"We have a lot of traveling and research to do, Kath," I concluded. "A lot of places to see and people to meet, and a baby such as you dreamed of would really mess things up."

"Sounds kind of selfish, don't you think?"

"No, I don't. We've earned these blessings, and now I believe it's time to enjoy them!"

What I was really saying, of course, was that I was too busy being "rich and famous," as my kids put it, to mess with other people's problem children. Which, when it comes down to it, *was* selfish. And extremely unrighteous, too. At the time, however, it didn't feel that way at all.

"Blaine," Kathy continued, changing the subject just a little, "I think I should begin to look for her."

"And I don't," I said, feeling more and more irritated. "I'm telling you, Kath, that would ruin our lifestyle, and I'm not about to let that happen!"

For a moment or two my wife was silent. The room was somewhat lighter, and the birds in the sycamore trees outside our window were warming to their dawn chorus. Everything had seemed so peaceful, so promising in our lives. Now this!

"I can see," Kathy said, her voice suddenly quiet, "that Heavenly Father is going to have to humble you."

To Kathy, God is truly her Heavenly Father—a loving Deity she can approach at any time, for any reason, and receive a kind and warm reception. Some people call this faith, but for Kathy it has simply been reality.

"What?" I groused. "*Humble* me? I already am humble! I just—"

"I saw our little girl," Kathy said, stopping me in mid-sentence. "I know it, and I know we're supposed to have her. But she won't come as long as you feel this way. So, starting this morning, I think we should pray that she will come. I'm going to, anyway. And I'm also going to pray that you will be humbled enough to accept her and love her."

I probably should have been terrified by Kathy's pronouncement, for long experience has taught me that she usually gets what she prays for. Unfortunately, I paid no attention to her. I went on my merry way, blissfully ignoring the faith she was exercising in my behalf. After all, it seemed I could do no wrong in my affairs, and my opinions were highly valued and sought after by others. Surely, I thought, I would be right about this dream baby as well.

As it turned out, however, the Lord not only heard Kathy's prayers but sided with her in her opinion of my humility—or lack thereof. In confirmation, he provided a second witness. Shortly after Kathy's dream, my mother called to tell us that she had also had a dream in which she had seen Kathy presenting me with a new little baby. "But," she warned sternly, "you will not get this child unless your family is better prepared for her—more righteous and spiritual."

"Thanks, Mom," I said, stifling a yawn. "We're trying to teach them, but you know how kids are these days—"

Now, with my perfect 20/20 hindsight, I truly wish I had paid attention to these two women, for life rather quickly began getting harder. Besides the normal horrors that came with trying to help guide our children through their teenage angst, I began making some foolish business decisions. I went deeply into debt on a speculative venture, mortgaging to the hilt every asset I had and hoping against hope that it would all work out. It didn't. Within two years of Kathy's dream and the commencement of her prayers, through no fault of anyone but myself, I had lost everything in this world except my family and my pride. And six months later, still being battered by the world, I could see that my family was reeling and even my pride was starting to waver.

"Are you still praying for me to get humbled?" I moaned at my wife one night near the end of 1985.

"Every day." She smiled sweetly.

"Well, knock it off, will you? If I get any more humble, it's going to kill me!"

"Or save you. Are you ready for our little girl yet?"

"Kath—"

"I mean it, Blaine. She's a special baby, and the Lord will not send her to our home until we are spiritually ready for her." Abruptly her look softened. "But don't feel so bad, hon. You're not the only one being humbled. The Lord is working his miracle on all of us, the kids and me included. More and more I have the feeling that our little girl is truly going to be an angel from heaven, and the Lord wants us all to be ready when she comes."

"You really think she's going to come?"

"I do!" Kathy was clearly convinced, and doubting her was becoming more and more difficult.

"And you also think we're changing?"

"Well, we're certainly not perfect, if that's what you mean." Kathy smiled again. "But I do see some promising signs."

"Such as?"

"Such as not so much fighting between the kids."

"Or us?" I asked hopefully.

"That, too. Family prayers are more regular and feel more meaningful. I know my personal prayers have changed, and I think yours have too. Our family Bible study is more regular, the kids' grades in school are going up, and we're watching less TV. I'd say those are all positive changes."

As I thought about it, I had to agree. Lately, because I had been literally forced to my knees, I had found myself constantly repenting before the Lord of the sins—both big and little—that I seemed to slip into so easily. More significantly, I was actually starting to get answers to my own prayers—feelings and impressions that gave me a little greater understanding of certain things. Those changes were amazing to me, for I had been trying to change for years and had never pulled it off.

My writing was also changing, growing more sober, more difficult, maybe even more honest. Harsh circumstances were forcing me to face myself more squarely, seeking, pondering, probing, asking, praying, feeling, acknowledging not only embarrassing weaknesses but occasional wonderful attributes that I had never dared hope might exist.

Such changes in myself were surprising. But what really amazed me were my children. Three or four times in the past few months I hadn't been able to scrape enough money together to pay the utilities or car payment. Each time, my older kids had willingly chipped in entire paychecks from their part-time jobs and paid the bills for me. (Is that humbling enough?) And in the most destitute yet memorable Christmas of my life, I had tearfully watched my family open sweet and thoughtful gifts from an unknown Santa Claus who turned out (why was I surprised?) to be my own children—the teenagers I had thought a year or two before were going to heck in a handbasket.

Well, at least one of us had been—

FOSTER CHILDREN

"See? I knew you would love them!"

"How could anybody love anything this tiny?" I grumbled, cradling the newborn infant in my arms. Of course I was teasing, for I was amazed at how easy it was to cuddle this little boy whom I'd never even heard of until the day before.

"I don't know why," Kathy continued as she mixed formula and warmed the baby's bottle, "but I couldn't get rid of the feeling that we needed to become foster parents."

"I sort of thought they'd come a little bigger."

"I told you I signed up for the newborns. I feel like we have to do this, Blaine, before we can obtain the little girl the Lord has promised us."

As I watched my wife, filled with wonder at her tenacity, I realized she might very well be right. But even if she weren't, I was very much enjoying these little children who were coming to stay with us a week or so before going on to their adoptive homes.

Those were wonderful times as our foster children passed one after another through our home. As I held and cuddled and helped nurture those tiny little people with their various problems and their different skin colors, I came to see how wrong I had been. I absolutely loved those children, every single one of them! I loved them as much as I loved my own, and it made not a particle of difference that other people had been their parents.

Our own children felt the same, excitedly taking turns giving each new child a temporary name. We named one little girl Stephanie after a neighbor one of our sons had a crush on, and a tiny, bellowing boy we named Justin—Chief Justin, we called him, of the Supreme Court. Our children loved them all, held them, fed and changed them, got up at night with them sometimes when we were too tired, and wept with my wife and me each time one of them left our home to begin his or her new life elsewhere. Yet the weeping was joyful, too, for we all knew "our" babies were on to bigger and better things with families all their own.

But while we watched other families being blessed, our own little girl failed to appear. Social Services, in approving us for foster care, had stated emphatically that foster families were never considered for adoption. We had agreed to that and so never looked for our little girl to be among our foster babies. We simply waited while we cared for those sweet children who were going to bless the lives of others, convinced that our own divinely appointed daughter was coming, but leaving her manner of arrival, as well as the timing of it, up to the Lord.

And then I had a dream.

"Kath," I said as early one morning as I could force open my eyes, "I think I saw her."

"Who?"

I gave an exaggerated sigh. "Who? Who are you always talking about? I think I saw our little girl."

Rolling over, Kathy looked at me skeptically. "Really?"

"Well, it was my turn, you know. I mean, if the Lord is going to give everybody else in this family dreams—"

Kathy smiled patiently. "So what did you see?"

"I saw Nate holding a tiny baby girl on the couch in the family room. I think it means she'll be coming sometime after he gets home from Arizona next spring. Let's see, that will be May of 1988. So expect your little baby sometime after that."

"Like a month?" Kathy's smile turned mischievous. "Or a year? Or maybe a decade? Are you really even sure it was her?"

And because I wasn't, and because I can hardly bear wives who persecute their perfectly wonderful husbands, my only defense was to grab her ribs and start tickling.

OUR ANGEL FINALLY COMES

"Kathy, telephone," I called, then idly balanced the receiver on my shoulder while I waited for my wife to pick up the phone in the kitchen. It was Wednesday, August 31, 1988. Nate had been home three months and had already moved into an apartment with some friends, and I was at my easel, painting an illustration to be used as the cover for one of my books.

The woman on the line had sounded familiar, sort of like Sharon, the woman who had overseen our efforts as a foster family. But it had been nearly a year since our last baby, and we had assumed that that period of our lives had concluded. A good thing, too, I thought a little grimly, for our financial "humbling" had continued, bringing with it the loss of our home. Now we were in the middle of packing and look- ing around for a home to rent—a mission that was feeling more and more impossible. Not a good time, I thought, to be taking in any new foster babies.

Kathy said hello, and I was not surprised to hear the woman iden- tify herself as Sharon. Normally I would have hung up at that point, but for some reason I felt like eavesdropping and left the phone on my shoulder.

"Kathy," Sharon asked, "are you available to take another foster baby?"

"Of course," Kathy replied without any hesitation. "When?"

"Probably tomorrow. I'll call you."

"Sounds wonderful. Is it a boy or a girl?"

"She's a darling little girl. Uh . . . you might have her a little longer than the usual week or so. Will that be a problem?"

"I don't think so. Why? Is something the matter?"

"Well, she has some health problems. She's hydrocephalic, and she was born without a cortex. It may take us a while to find an adoptive family. If we don't find one, we'll probably have to place her in an institution."

Hydrocephalic and no cortex, I thought as I listened in. It sounded serious, though truthfully I had no clue what those things meant.

"Well, don't worry," I suddenly realized my wife was saying. "If you can't find anybody to adopt her, we will!"

"What!" my mind screamed into the silence that hung between Kathy and Sharon, completely blocking out Kathy's dream of a little girl who was being rushed to a hospital. What was she thinking? Didn't we have enough problems already? Did we have to go around volunteering to take on more? She was crazy! And besides that, she—

"You would do that?" Sharon was asking, her voice incredulous.

"Of course we would. She deserves a family as much as anyone, doesn't she?"

My mind spinning with the magnitude of what Kathy had just offered to do, I listened as Sharon thanked her and promised to call the next day. Carefully then I hung up and made a beeline for the stairs. Moments later Kathy and I were seated across from each other in the kitchen.

"Do you have any idea . . ." I started to demand, and then I noticed her tears. "Kath, what is it?"

"I . . . I don't know," she stammered, her voice little more than a whisper. "I had the . . . strangest feeling when Sharon was talking to me. Blaine, I think this little girl is *our baby.*"

"What?" For the first time in months those memories of her dream, as well as my own, came back to me. "Our baby?"

"Uh-huh. Remember how I was hurrying her to a hospital?"

"Well, sure, but—"

"Blaine, I think this is her! That's why I said what I did about adopting her. I know foster parents aren't supposed to adopt, or even to request it. But the feeling that she is to be ours was so strong, I just couldn't help it!"

For a moment I was silent, digesting Kathy's news. "Do you know what Sharon was talking about—the things that are wrong with the baby?"

Kathy shook her head. "Not exactly. I'm pretty sure hydrocephalus is water on the brain. I remember reading that somewhere. And I think the cortex is a membrane, though I'm not certain where it is. But it won't matter, not any more than the fact that we're foster parents. If this little girl is the baby we've seen in our dreams, then Heavenly Father is going to see that we have her, no matter what."

"Kids," Kathy declared that night at supper, "we're getting a new baby tomorrow."

"Serious?" fifteen-year-old Dan asked. It was interesting to see how much he loved babies. It was a wonderful quality I would never have known about had we not entered the foster parent program. "Boy or girl?"

"She's a little girl," Kathy replied.

"*Yes!*" thirteen-year-old Michelle shouted as she clenched her fist triumphantly. "Finally, after all those goofy boys!"

"Boys aren't goofy!" Dan declared heatedly. I should say that Dan and Michelle had been arguing since even before Michelle had learned how to talk, and we had tried every way that we knew to stop them. I had even turned them over to God, as Kathy had done with me. Apparently they were even harder cases than I, though, for we hadn't seen any significant progress yet.

"Oh, yeah?" This was Michelle again, defiant as ever. "You try changing boys' diapers and see how you like getting squirted!"

Travis, eighteen and also a connoisseur of good arguments, smiled but amazingly did not enter into the conversation, which I considered fortunate. Travis, too, was affected by the babies. But he didn't like the pain when they left, so he tried to avoid having much contact with them.

"We may need a little extra help with this one," Kathy continued. "She has what I think is water on the brain, and she's missing a membrane somewhere. Whatever, it's serious enough that Sharon might not find a family right away. May we count on your help?"

Soberly the kids nodded.

"Mom, is this *our* baby?" Dan asked abruptly.

Kathy shook her head. "I don't know, Danny. I suppose she might be. But whether she is or not, let's remember to pray for the baby's health, and to ask Heavenly Father to see to it that she goes to the right family. Okay?"

Again the kids nodded soberly. And I was probably the most sober one of all.

The next day Kathy drove to the Social Services office and returned with the baby. I will never forget my first sight of her. At two days of age she was tiny, less than five pounds, and as I took her I remember thinking that I could easily have held her in one hand. She had lots of dark hair, her dark eyes were wide open, and, so far as I could tell, everything about her was perfect. I even examined her tiny head for signs of swelling from too much fluid, but I could find none at all. Except for a slightly recessed forehead, she seemed perfect to me, absolutely beautiful, and I thought that if she wasn't ours, somebody else was surely going to be blessed.

"Well, little one," I asked as I cradled her in my arms, "are you the baby girl we've been waiting for all these years?"

Her only answer was a little fussing and kicking, which served to get her hoisted away and into the anxious arms of Michelle. A small bottle plopped into her mouth silenced her at least temporarily, giving Kathy and me a moment to talk.

"Now that you've seen her," I asked after we had made our way upstairs into my office, "what do you think?"

Kathy smiled. "I think she's our daughter, Blaine. I really do."

"Why?"

"I don't know. Just a feeling, I guess. Besides, she looks like her, though I don't remember her being this tiny."

"Maybe in your dream she was a little older. Did you learn any more from Sharon?"

"Only that she wants to take her to Primary Children's Medical Center in Salt Lake City for some tests."

"What kind of tests?"

"I don't know. She didn't say."

"So, can we adopt her?"

"Well, Sharon says the agency is considering us. What they do is run a computer search through all the families in America that have been approved for adoption. If no one else wants her, they'll consider alternatives such as us."

Slowly I shook my head. "We'll never get her, then," I said, feeling unaccountably sad. "She's so cute that thousands of families will want her!"

"Honey," Kathy said as she reached for my hand, "just have faith. If she is meant to be a part of our family, it will work out just fine."

Kathy was right and I knew it, but the odds against it seemed so high that I didn't even dare hope. And I wanted to hope in the worst way, for suddenly, after having held her at most for five minutes, I wanted this little girl to be my daughter. It made no sense at all, but I did. I was head over heels in love with her. That night, as we sent our petitions heavenward, mine was one of the most fervent pleas of all.

The next day, quite by accident, we learned the nature of our baby's "missing membrane." One of our friends, a nurse at a hospital in a neighboring community, dropped by to visit with Kathy. When Kathy told her we had a new foster baby, she began waxing eloquent over a tiny baby who had been born at her hospital a couple of days before.

"She was so cute!" she exclaimed. "Even though she didn't have a brain, she was the most alert baby in the nursery, holding her head up and looking around just like she knew what she was doing. Everyone fell in love with her. If I could have adopted her, I'd have done it in a minute!"

The conversation drifted to other things, but, as our friend was leaving, Kathy took her in to see "our" baby.

"Why," she exclaimed with surprise, "that's her! That's the baby girl I was telling you about—the one without a brain."

"She doesn't have a brain?" Kathy asked, astounded. "But . . . how can she live?"

Margie smiled. "Well, she does have a brain stem. It runs the autonomic nervous system. All babies use it exclusively when they are first born, which is why this child seems so normal. In six weeks or so, when she would normally begin to shift functions into the cortex, or the two hemispheres of her brain, this little girl will start having problems. It isn't likely that she will live long after that."

After the kids had all gone to bed, Kathy and I talked late into the night, thinking, wondering, probing each other's feelings. This was a whole different situation than we had anticipated and dreamed of, and neither of us knew exactly what to do or how to feel. We thought we could deal with health problems. But such a terrible and permanent disability seemed overwhelming, as did the possibility of so soon a death.

The next morning we lay in each other's arms, continuing to share our feelings about the tiny child in the bassinet across the room. Despite her massive problems, both of us continued to feel that this was the child we had seen in our dreams, the celestial little girl the Lord had promised to send us and for whose reception our family had been trying to prepare. With God's help, we were beginning to believe that we could somehow take care of her.

Now, if only the Lord would also tell the folks at Social Services that we were the family—

HEAVEN REVEALS A NAME

"Look at this, everybody. This is amazing!" A couple of days had passed, and Kathy had been making a batch of cookies while the rest of us were finishing breakfast and getting ready for school and work. Sharon had not yet arrived to take the baby to the hospital, which was that day's task, and she was lying quietly in a car seat on the counter, already fitting in as part of our family.

"What is it?" I asked, getting up to see what Kathy was so excited about.

"These cookies. This child's entire head is smaller than one of these cookies! I can't get over how tiny she is."

"She's little, all right," I said as I leaned over and kissed her forehead. "Little, and cute!"

"What are we going to name her?" Dan was always concerned about names for our babies.

"Any ideas?"

Two or three names were tossed about, but somehow none of them felt right.

"I have a suggestion," Kathy said. "Since she's Heavenly Father's special child, why don't we have Dad pray and ask what God would want her to be named."

"Kath," I responded, feeling uneasy with such a burden, "I don't—"

"Yeah, Dad," Travis said as he piled the dishes in the sink. "You're the father here, so it should be your responsibility to at least find out if God cares what she's named."

"He'll care," Michelle interjected. "God always cares!"

Dan walked over and took the baby's tiny hand between his fingers. "I don't really care what we name her," he said as he gazed tenderly at her, "just so long as it isn't one of those dumb names out of the Bible."

"Danny!"

"Well, knowing Dad," he replied defensively as he grabbed his books and headed for the door, "that's probably what he'll come up with. Jezebel or Hepzibah or something else just as stupid."

Ducking to avoid the slipper I threw at him, he grinned and was gone. A little later, after Sharon had come and taken the baby, I was alone on my knees in my bedroom, Dan's words ringing in my ears as I asked prayerfully about a name for the little girl I was positive would be our daughter.

For some time as I prayed, I was finding it difficult to focus. Worries about the child's health, about how we would take care of her while we were moving, how we would afford the medical expenses I knew would come with her—these concerns and many more swirled around and around in my mind. Yet again and again I came back in prayer to the issue of her name, pleading to know if the Lord had a name he wanted us to call her.

Gradually I realized that a passage of scripture was bouncing around in my head, a passage from the New Testament. Thinking of Dan's admonition, I pushed the idea aside, only to find it there again moments later. Finally, with a sigh of resignation, I got up and walked to the nightstand, picked up the Bible, and for a change turned right to the verses I had been considering. Beginning at verse four of

1 Corinthians 13, I read: "Charity suffereth long, and is kind; charity envieth not; charity vaunteth not itself, is not puffed up. Doth not behave itself unseemly, seeketh not her own, is not easily provoked, thinketh no evil; rejoiceth not in iniquity, but rejoiceth in the truth; beareth all things, believeth all things, hopeth all things, endureth all things. Charity never faileth."

Slowly I read the verses again, somehow knowing even as I read them that these words perfectly described our little girl. More, I also felt certain that the Lord wanted her to be named Charity.

"Charity?" Kathy responded a little later when I showed her the scripture. "I like that name. It fits her. She certainly is a patient little thing. And if she doesn't have a brain, she'll never think evil thoughts or rejoice in iniquity."

"Or be puffed up with her own importance," I added, remembering too vividly my own past struggles. "But I had some interesting feelings while I was praying, Kath. I felt again that she is to be our daughter."

Kathy smiled.

"But more than that, the thought came to me that this is not a current decision, if that makes any sense. I'm not sure I understand this, and I could never say if this were true for anyone else, but I believe that all of us, including Charity, agreed to be a family long before any of us were born. And so it's going to happen, no matter how many families want her."

"Well, you know what I've been feeling—"

"It will happen. But Kath, I also had the feeling that Charity willingly accepted her birth defect, in part, at least, because it would help her come to us. In spite of that," and suddenly I found my eyes tearing up, "she is an incredibly righteous and powerful soul with a brilliant and active mind. It doesn't matter what handicaps having no physical brain will bring. I feel that she will always be aware of us and of what is transpiring around her. The Lord has not simply abandoned her here with no means of communicating with either him or us. Through the power of the Holy Spirit I believe she will do both."

"Do you mean something like angels visiting her?"

I grinned. "Yeah, something like that. It'd be great having a bunch of real angels hanging around here, wouldn't it?"

That evening when the family was gathered together, I read the scripture and told of my feeling about naming our little girl Charity.

"I don't like it," Michelle said bluntly. "Like Danny said, it's a Bible name."

"Well, at least it isn't a dumb one," Dan replied easily.

"I think it's dumb. And I think you ought to go back and pray again, Dad. I think Heavenly Father ought to give us a choice."

"Are you serious?" I asked.

"Yes," she replied, and I could tell that she was. "Go do it right now, before we go to bed. I want a choice."

Looking at my wife for help, I found none, only a smile and a slight shrug of her shoulders. So, with a sigh of resignation, I headed again for the bedroom, certain that no inspiration would come.

Apparently, however, God was as concerned about Michelle's feelings as he was about the baby's name, for almost instantly I felt to get my Bible and read it again. I did so, finishing Paul's chapter I had started earlier, and as the Holy Spirit again bore witness I found myself chuckling.

"Did you get an answer already?" Michelle asked, surprised at my sudden reappearance.

"I did!" I smiled. "And you were right. We have a choice—actually, of three names."

"Really?" Michelle was very excited.

"Uh-huh."

"Well," Kathy asked, as interested as any of the kids, "what are they?"

Still smiling, I held up the Bible and looked at Michelle. "It says right here, 'And now abideth faith, hope, charity, these three.' You decide, Sis."

"Faith or Hope?" Michelle rolled her eyes in disgust. "Those aren't choices! They're worse than Charity."

"Those are the three names I think God gave me."

"Well," she declared with an exaggerated sigh, "then I guess I have to pick Charity."

"So did the Apostle Paul," I pointed out to her. "Right here, he says Charity is the greatest of the three."

"Really?" she asked innocently, and then we all laughed together. Suddenly she jumped to her feet. "I vote that we make Charity's middle name Afton, after Grandma Wagstaff. All in favor raise their hands."

We all did. Our little girl now had a name: Charity Afton. We just didn't know if it would ever become official.

WE MAKE A COMMITMENT

◆───

The tests conducted at Primary Children's Medical Center confirmed what our friend Margie had told us—little Charity Afton had no brain. The medical term for her problem was hydranencephaly. In a letter to Sharon dated September 2, 1988 (which we did not see until I was preparing this manuscript), Dr. Marion L. Walker, chairman of pediatric neurosurgery at PCMC, wrote:

> Her CT scan demonstrates severe brain loss in the supratentorial compartment. She has some occipital lobes bilaterally and normal appearing basal ganglia, thalamus, brain stem and posterior fossa. She essentially has no visible temporal, parietal or frontal brain. There is no indication in this CT scan to suggest increased intracranial pressure.
>
> IMPRESSION: 1. Severe developmental anomaly. 2. Severe loss of brain substance bilaterally secondary to probable intrauterine stroke.
>
> This patient has very little potential for development beyond the infant stage. With almost complete loss of supratentorial brain, she has essentially no chance of developing beyond infant skills. Children with this much brain damage rarely survive childhood. Although some may live four to five years or possibly

longer, it is unusual for these children to live beyond eighteen months.

As Sharon explained to us the day after the tests and examination, the doctors had told her that Charity would be unable to enjoy any of her senses. She wouldn't be able to see, hear, feel, taste, or smell. She would know nothing of what was going on around her, would never have any control over any part of her body, would never experience or be able to express joy, happiness, and love. She would simply live her life in a vegetative state. Her immune system would be pretty much nonexistent, causing her to contract practically every disease and illness that came along, especially colds and flu. And she would very likely die in the near future from pneumonia.

On the plus side (if these could be called pluses), the doctors had said Charity wouldn't grow very much or get very heavy, she would never feel any pain, and she wouldn't have to endure this life for very long.

"Do these things matter to you?" Sharon asked us.

"No," Kathy replied firmly, "not at all. If she needs a home, we'll be happy to give it to her."

I gulped and nodded in agreement.

"Very well." Sharon smiled. "As soon as we know something, I'll let you know. By the way, she was so darling there at the hospital. She didn't fuss at all, but held her head up and just seemed to watch what was going on. She's really an amazing little girl."

"We know," I said as I took Kathy's hand. "We think she's an angel."

"Yes," Sharon replied as she moved out the door, "I believe she is."

"If Charity doesn't have a brain," Travis asked one night after he came home from work, "can she really be alive?"

His question stunned us. "Do you believe she isn't alive?" I asked.

"I didn't say that. I think she's as alive as we are. But other people don't feel like that, including a guy at my work. He was being a real jerk about it."

"Did you tell him about Charity?"

"Yeah, but I guess maybe I shouldn't have. He thinks we should just let her starve to death. 'Sure,' I told him. 'Just murder her and then go have lunch.' He's a major pain."

"A kid in school said the same thing," Dan piped in. "I told him if she was breathing and her heart was beating, that made her alive."

"So, what happened?"

"Nothing. He knew I was right, so he shut up."

"Well," Travis said, looking exasperated and abruptly switching sides, "maybe you weren't right. If she has no brain to think with, how can she be alive or have consciousness? If you don't let religion into the conversation, that's a darn good question."

"Yeah, but religion has to play a part, too."

"Why?" Travis was enjoying this.

"Because we believe in it!" Dan growled.

"All right," I said, stepping in to referee, "just exactly how does religion answer the problem?"

Both boys looked at each other. "Because of her spirit," Dan replied first. "Paul says that God is the Father or Creator of our spirits, and, like the bumper sticker says, God don't make no mistakes."

"What do you mean?" I pressed, both surprised and pleased by Dan's response.

"He means," Travis interjected, "that despite the fact that they have no physical brains, and no matter how long they may live, from eighteen seconds to thirty years or more, babies like Charity are born with whole or perfect spirits. They have minds, they have consciousness, and despite their handicaps they are as much human beings as those who, say, happen to be born without arms or legs."

"Or even if they're born 'whole' like us," Dan added. "Isn't that right, Dad?"

I told them that I thought it was. As far as I was concerned, little Charity was as alive as any of us because her spirit was as whole as ours. And time, I felt, would prove us right.

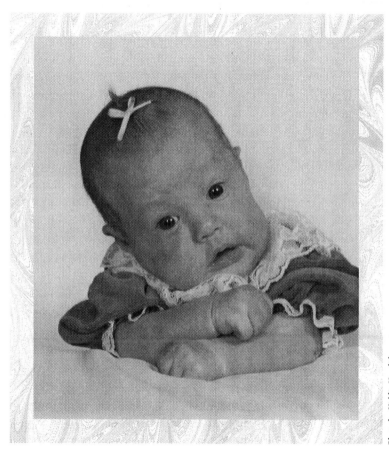

Charity at six weeks of age.

THE BIRTH FAMILY DECIDES

"Honey, Sharon called." Kathy sounded concerned. "The birth family wants to take Charity again."

"Why?" I asked. "What's going on?"

"I guess they're having a hard time letting go." She sat down at the end of my desk, and I noticed for the first time how drawn and tired she looked. Charity had not been sleeping well, and because we were a little older than we had been when our other children were tiny, we were both feeling the strain.

"I don't really blame them," she said, massaging her forehead. "If I was her mother or grandmother, I couldn't bear letting Charity go. I think I'd rather die."

"I think it would be just as difficult for the men in her family," I pointed out.

"I'm sure you're right. Sharon says they're going to keep her at least through the weekend. She . . . uh . . . she says some of the family are considering placing her in an institution so they can visit her when they want."

"Seriously?"

"Well, that's what I've been told. Would you mind giving Charity a blessing before she goes?"

I looked at Kathy quizzically, thinking of the process of laying on of hands in prayer that was a part of our religious belief. "I guess so. What for?"

"So she can somehow communicate to the birth family that she is supposed to be our little girl."

Well, I am a believer in the Lord Jesus Christ and his infinite power, but that is not always the same as having faith in him. "Can I do that with a blessing?" I asked doubtfully.

Kathy smiled and rose to her feet. "*You* probably can't. But the Lord can do anything he wants. So if you'll pronounce the blessing, then the Lord can take over and bring her back to us. Sharon said she will be here in about thirty minutes, so when you're ready—"

I gave the blessing, and for the next three days we worried ourselves silly. Or at least I did. At last, however, Sharon returned with our little angel, bearing also the news that the birth family had finally felt peace about placing her for adoption.

As Sharon handed Charity to me, our three-week-old little girl burst into a radiant smile that did not go away for more than thirty minutes. Though she was not supposed to be able to feel emotions or even to smile, she obviously could, and we were awed by it. As we basked in her smile's glow, we knew that Charity knew she was home!

THE WORST DAY OF KATHY'S LIFE

The day Charity came home to us, September 12, 1988, Social Services called and informed us that a computer search of the entire country had failed to turn up even one interested family. Therefore, if we were still interested, we could proceed with first qualifying for and then hopefully completing the adoption. Needless to say, our home rang that night with the joy of knowing our family would now be complete.

Unfortunately, the announcement also signaled the beginning of some real difficulties, both for Charity and for us. By the next day Charity was crying more than usual, and within a very few days she was crying almost continually. Examining her ourselves, we felt certain that her head was swelling, and this was confirmed by our pediatrician, who for the first time thought he also heard a heart murmur.

Charity continued to cry and tremble with pain until October 5, when in desperation we took her to the Primary Children's Medical Center. There we met for the first time Dr. Marion Walker, and he confirmed that her head was indeed enlarging. We appreciated his advice and his tender approach, and felt relieved when he said he still hoped to avoid surgery to place a shunt, but that we should come back in two weeks for further evaluation.

Although Charity seemed to do a little better in the next two weeks, our lives were truly coming apart. Not only were we in the throes of the business failure that was forcing us to move from our home, but Kathy's physical health was starting to deteriorate. She'd had back problems off and on for years, but now they were coming back with alarming regularity, and there was no medical consensus on what was wrong. Worse, her father had grown desperately ill, and she was feeling torn between spending time with her parents and caring for our struggling little infant.

"Well, folks," Dr. Walker said after his follow-up examination, "Charity's head is definitely enlarging. I would imagine she is becoming more irritable, too."

"She is," Kathy acknowledged. "She's been doing a lot of crying, and a lot of trembling because of pain."

"Technically she isn't supposed to feel pain, you know."

"Well, we don't feel that Charity is a technicality. She's definitely in pain, and we know it."

Dr. Walker smiled. "I'm sure you're right. And she does respond to Tylenol, which would suggest the same conclusion. Changing the subject, I'd still rather avoid placing a shunt. There's a good chance this growth will stop and she will stabilize. Shall we try another two weeks and see her again?"

The next few weeks were agonizing, as Charity grew steadily worse. It was just as well we had decided to wait, though, for we knew we had to move out of our home right away. Fortunately we had located a home we could rent, so at least there was some peace about where we would be going. On Monday, November 7, just as we began to move, both Charity and Kathy's father began to decline rapidly. The next day I watched my dear wife experience what was no doubt the most difficult day of her life—at least up until then.

"Honey, something's going wrong with her. I mean really wrong!"

I was holding our screaming daughter at the moment, trying unsuccessfully to comfort her. "I know, Kath," I admitted. "I'm sure it's her head, but she isn't even responding to Tylenol any more. Besides, the bottle's empty—"

"We have more, don't we?"

"Somewhere." I looked around at the shambles in the home we were moving into. We had now slept there one night, so at least our beds were in place. Unfortunately, everything else was goodness-only-knew-where. Our friend Max Walters had been hauling loads of boxes in his pickup truck—a terribly needed gesture of friendship—but because I had been so involved with Charity I had no idea where he had been putting things. But, I thought, I could at least look around—

The telephone rang, our first call in the new home, and as Kathy answered it I watched her face drain of color.

"Dad's dying," she said as she replaced the receiver, a stricken look on her face. "I need to be with Mom!"

Moments later, trying desperately to make arrangements so she could go to her father's side, Kathy grabbed a bite of something to eat and broke off a major portion of a tooth, exposing nerves and leaving a jagged edge that quickly cut the side of her tongue to shreds. We were searching for some sort of painkiller to deal with that, and trying to locate our dentist, when the phone rang again and the school informed us that Michelle had run a sewing-machine needle completely through her finger and was at the hospital, needing a ride home.

Because I couldn't leave Charity, we found a neighbor boy, Ryan Wooden, who could go pick up Michelle. Kathy managed to locate our dentist and have some temporary work done so she could go to her parents. Unfortunately, her father passed away before she could get there, which made her grief even harder to bear. And Charity cried all that night.

As I said, it truly was the worst day of my sweetheart's life. What we didn't understand was that it was simply a prelude to harder days to come.

An Inspired Lullaby

◆

Only a parent who has spent agonizing and sleepless nights with a sick child can know the feeling of helplessness it brings. There was a night, shortly after Dad's passing, that brought that home to me. Exhausted because of lack of sleep, Kathy and I were both in a dead stupor when, shortly after midnight, Charity began once again to scream from pain.

Asking Kathy to remain in bed, I arose and took our anguished little girl downstairs, where I alternately prayed and wept, doing anything and everything I could think of to relieve her suffering—all to no avail.

It seemed so strange to me, this anguish of my daughter's. We had been told she would never feel pain, yet obviously she was suffering almost more than she could bear. She was also growing at a normal rate, though she had been expected to remain small. And on the rare occasions when she felt well, she smiled and responded exactly as our other children had done. Was it possible, I wondered, that the doctors had been wrong about her?

I didn't know, and of course at that moment I didn't really care. All I wanted was for her to be made free of pain. So as I sat and rocked, or stood and paced, I prayed as fervently as I have ever prayed in my life, pleading that she be freed of the pain that seemed to be destroying her.

And then, sometime after three in the morning, I felt a great peace settle upon me, and as I wondered at it, the words and tune of a little lullaby began forming in my mind. Hesitantly I began to sing. To my amazement, Charity's crying stopped. With wide-open eyes she lay still in my arms, taking in every sound coming out of my mouth.

Though both the lyrics and tune were simple, Charity seemed to hang on every note, every word.

> *Oh Charity, pure Charity,*
> *Do you know who you are?*
> *Oh Charity, my Charity,*
> *An angel from afar.*
> *Our Father sent you to my home,*
> *For brief mortality.*
> *Oh Charity, smiling Charity,*
> *My Savior's gift of love to me.*

There were more verses than this, three more, describing my feelings about her pain, her becoming a part of our family, and her eternal destiny. Over and over I sang the verses, and as long as I was singing she was still, lying peacefully in my arms. I thought I had loved her before, but during those long hours we communed, spirit to spirit, and I truly felt of her sweet and perfect nature. She was indeed Christ's gift to me. I knew that with all my heart and soul, and suddenly I wanted more than I had ever wanted anything in my life to be worthy of her—and of him—when I finally left this vale of sorrow and tears.

Sometime near daybreak Charity finally fell asleep. A couple of hours later, after I had written down the lullaby and shared it with Kathy, she told me that a night or two earlier she, too, had been given a tender little song, one remarkably similar to mine, and it had had precisely the same effect. In listening, our little darling had somehow found peace and the courage to continue. And, in the face of her incredible courage, so had we.

THE FIRST SURGERY

◆

On November 17, 1988, when things had settled down a little at home, we took Charity back to PCMC, where Dr. Walker finally operated, performing a right ventriculoperitoneal shunt placement.

"Oh, Blaine," Kathy whispered in anguish when we saw our baby a couple of hours later, lying still but softly whimpering, "look at the poor little dear. Charity, Mommy's sorry—"

Charity did look awful. The right side of her head had been completely shaved of her beautiful hair, and her scalp was now covered with a red-orange substance that looked too much like blood to give me much peace.

"It's called Betadine," Dr. Walker said as he joined us. "It's a disinfectant. Charity tolerated the surgery quite well, but I thought you'd like to know exactly what we did."

"We would."

"All right. First we made an incision high on the side of her head, there under the bandage, and a burr hole was drilled through her skull. A ventricular catheter or shunt was inserted through the hole. The other end of the shunt was threaded beneath her skin down her neck and back, under her shoulder blade, around her side, and into her abdominal cavity. There a second incision was made to insure correct placement. If you look carefully, you can see the tube there beneath her skin."

"That's a major surgery, isn't it?" I asked as I gazed at the raised skin covering where the tube lay.

"It is, especially for a child this tiny. We expect that the shunt will now drain the excess fluid from Charity's cranial cavity, thus relieving the pressure that has been causing her such distress."

"What if it doesn't work?" Kathy asked.

"Then we'll do it again." Dr. Walker smiled. "But don't worry. She'll most likely be just fine. I believe Charity's room will be on Four West. I'll probably see you there later today."

That afternoon, following postoperative recovery, Charity was transferred to Four West, a wing on the fourth floor, and there Kathy and I were first introduced to the sorrow, and the magic, of Primary Children's Medical Center.

This was not the new, gleaming white structure that now carries the Primary Children's Medical Center name, but the old, red brick hospital that once graced the upper reaches of the Avenues in Salt Lake City. Fifty years before our time it must have seemed to the builders that it would always be spacious and modern. Yet by November of 1988, as my wife and I stood with our suffering daughter in her crowded room, the whole facility seemed woefully inadequate. There was no privacy—for us, nurses, doctors, or other patients; there was little room for more than one visitor per child; each room had at least two children as patients (and some four or five); the hallways were always crowded with extra equipment as well as scurrying personnel, ambulatory patients, and curious visitors. I was feeling put out by the whole of it, and was not looking for good in much of anything.

Charity was placed in a stainless steel crib in a cubicle of a room in which were two other cribs, each with a tiny and very ill occupant. There were also three chairs, usually occupied by the three mothers, and considerable monitoring equipment. There was space in the center, but only a very little, for the doctors and nurses to occupy as they bustled in and out of the room.

"We're exceptionally crowded right now," a nurse smiled as I looked in vain for a place to sit. "Otherwise there would be only two beds, and there would be more room." She smiled again, something I was to learn was a trademark of those wonderful people. "But if you'll give me a few minutes, I'll see if I can find you a chair."

I thanked her and leaned over the side of Charity's crib, trying not to look at the other infants and thus seem nosy or intrusive. The tube in our two-month-old daughter's nose was for oxygen, helping her to breathe until the shock of her surgery was past. The wires on her chest and back monitored her heart and respiratory functions, and were the source of the constant-sounding alarm. Her pathetic-looking, half-shaved head, the shaved part swabbed with orange Betadine, as well as the bandaged incisions there and on her tummy, spoke further of the terrible damage Charity's tiny body had sustained.

"What's wrong with your baby?" a very young woman asked from right behind me. And that was when I began to realize that most of the parents of PCMC patients were in their twenties or maybe early thirties—kids who seemed way too young to be facing such problems as their children were experiencing. Kathy and I were definitely the old people in that hospital.

"Shunt surgery," Kathy responded. "To drain the excess fluid from her head."

"Oh," the woman responded as she rose and moved beside me to gaze tenderly at our daughter. "Poor little thing. She looks so tiny and alone. How did it go?"

"We hope just fine," Kathy replied. "We haven't heard otherwise."

The woman smiled. "That's good. Did Dr. Walker do it?"

We nodded.

"Good. He's the best! Another of his patients, a sweet little boy down the hall, is in for his fiftieth shunt revision. He's such a neat little kid."

"What's the problem with your little girl?" I asked into the awkward silence that followed her statement.

"She was born with spina bifida. This is her fourth surgery. I'm Carol, my daughter's name is Alyse, and this," she said, indicating the third mother in the room, "is Mary Ann. Yesterday her daughter Heather had surgery for a blocked colon. She's not quite two weeks old."

"Hi," Mary Ann said timidly.

We responded, and from that moment those three women were fast friends, bonded by their close proximity and the pain of their children. By the next day, we were also friends with the doctors and nurses who filed through the door of Charity's room. Most were extremely personable, and it didn't take us long to realize that we had become part of a big and constantly changing family, all of whom seemed as concerned about our little Charity as we were.

I also watched in awe as Kathy began reaching out to the other mothers, tenderly lifting their burdens and shouldering their pain with them. Within a day or so she knew the names of almost every mother—and child—on Four West. In spite of her sorrow over our own little child's suffering, she visited with the others, wept with them, hugged and held them, and somehow found time and strength to sit with them when crises came. And yet never for a minute did she neglect or forget our daughter.

Often over the next few days I strolled the halls or sat in the crowded waiting room, giving the doctors and nurses space and trying to divert my mind from Charity's pain. Always there were parents or grandparents in the waiting room, visiting, sleeping, or just staring off into space, too numb from their experience to do anything else. And there were children everywhere, for PCMC was a place for children.

"Kath," I muttered the next day as we walked down the hall toward the elevator, "I can hardly bear to look at these children. It . . . it hurts too much."

Kathy squeezed my hand. "I know, hon. You've never been able to handle seeing people hurting."

"Who could? Especially here, where the ones doing the hurting are innocent little people who don't even understand what's happening to them. I don't care if my kids do tease me about crying too easily. When I'm here, it's all I can do to keep myself from bawling all day long!"

And it was difficult. But how could we be expected to control our feelings of sympathy and sorrow when all about us were the maimed and tormented little bodies of children? There were children with cancer who had lost all their hair and strength to radiation and chemotherapy; accident victims who had lost limbs, eyesight, and so forth; victims of abuse who had suffered horrid injustices; children like little Charity who had struggled with problems from birth; and children ravaged by various terrible diseases. I could hardly bear to look at them, let alone begin to comprehend their pain.

Yet unfailingly the personnel at PCMC approached their tragic tasks with smiles and joyful attitudes, doing everything in their power to ease the pain and lift the burdens of the children. To that end, the wallpaper and even the little gowns and pajamas were bright and ani-mated. Some hospital personnel wore funny hats and teased the chil-dren into rare smiles and laughter. The nurses were unendingly cheer-ful. Ronald McDonald the clown was a regular visitor who always brought forth wide-eyed stares and giggles. And volunteer grandmas and grandpas came and sat for hours with children whose parents, for one reason or another, could not be there. In spite of the pain and suf-fering, it was truly a place of love and giving, and each night as Kathy and I lay exhausted but sleepless, discussing the day's events, our con-versation would always return to the magic of PCMC that we were feeling.

A Personality Becomes Evident

⁂ "Can you believe it, Blaine? Look at all these darling little out-fits. I think every woman in the neighborhood came to the shower."

Like Kathy, I was amazed at the outpouring of love and concern shown us by our friends and neighbors once Charity was home from the hospital. Knowing we had grown past the "new baby" stage of life, these dear people had responded to the news of our adopting a little girl by setting us up with baby clothing, a stroller, and all sorts of baby things that are only thought of once they're needed.

More, one after another these women had held our daughter and exclaimed at the powerful spirit of love and joy she seemed to radiate.

"I find it so amazing the way she affects people," Kathy said that night. "It's just like in my dream—person after person stopping me to see and hold Charity and feel her spirit."

"Why not, Kath? We feel that way ourselves." And we did, too. None of the kids seemed able to get enough of holding her, cuddling her, playing and laughing with her. I was the worst of the lot—I simply couldn't stop nuzzling and loving her, and I thrived on being in her presence.

What was most amazing to me, though, was her personality. She loved to be held and cuddled, she fussed if she didn't get her bottle on time, she enjoyed taking baths, and more and more her radiant smile was becoming a sought-after reward by all of us. The kids danced with her, made funny little noises in her ear, tickled her and bounced her on their knees, bundled her up and took her for walks in the stroller, and showed her off at every opportunity. And Kathy and I were constantly singing to her: Kathy sweet lullabies and hymns, and me strange little tunes that I made up on the spot, either telling her how I felt about her or sharing what was going on with the other members of the family. I took a lot of heat from the kids over those songs, but Charity seemed to enjoy them, and that was what counted most.

Of course, that meant she was hearing us, one of the senses we had expected her not to have. Not only could she hear, she could obviously hear well! No matter how quiet we tried to be, she could always tell when one of us was near. And she visibly reacted to external sounds. For instance, she loved music (the real kind, rather than my singing), but only certain types. She tolerated Neil Diamond and his music only if the kids were dancing with her to it. Otherwise, no thank you. She hated all other types of rock and roll and would stress out and actually become ill if she heard very much of it. She did not like country western (my own favorite at the time), and most classical music was stressful to her. On the other hand, she enjoyed children's songs—especially if children were singing them—certain numbers from Walt Disney, and all hymns. And of the hymns, the only ones she would ever coo along with were hymns written specifically about the Lord Jesus.

Over and over we watched these reactions of hers, which never varied, and the only conclusion we could ever reach was that she had brought her musical tastes intact from the realms above. After that, we all began thinking a little more about the kinds of music *we* enjoyed.

And we weren't the only ones who recognized Charity's distinct

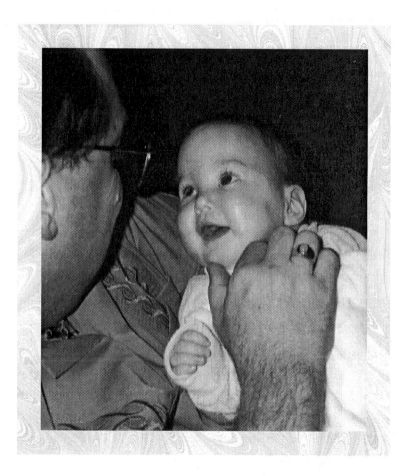

Three-month-old Charity gives her daddy a big smile.

personality. Mary Bushman, a county infant development nurse who helped us with Charity, described one of her visits to our home: "Charity was a beautiful baby with bright, huge blue eyes and a lovely, perfect body—no visible sign whatsoever of her handicap. She was always clean and sweet-smelling and obviously adored by her family. But she was different from any other child I ever visited, not only by her diagnosis but by her powerful presence. I had a most unusual feeling as I handled her and interacted with her—as though I was not talking to an infant but to a mature spirit-personality.

"One day as Kathy and I were observing and assessing Charity's condition, Blaine popped his head around the door frame and called to Charity. Her head turned instantly, her eyes focused on him as he came toward her, she smiled—and I was shocked. This little girl had no brain and so could not hear, could not see, and certainly could not focus. Those things were physically impossible for her. And yet—

"Later that day I had an appointment with a doctor whom I trusted completely and for whom I had the highest respect. I related to him my experience with Charity and Blaine, thinking that perhaps there had been a flaw in my research or something I didn't understand about her condition. He shook his head and said there was no medical explanation. 'Of course what you witnessed is impossible with her diagnosis,' he continued. 'Medical science has confirmed that. What you witnessed, therefore, had to be accomplished by the power of her spirit.'"

Charity's spirit was indeed very strong, and it was wonderful to have her feeling better after her surgery. That was all we could have asked for—or so we thought, until suddenly she got her days and nights mixed up.

"Maybe if I were younger," I grumbled at about 2:30 on Thanksgiving morning, "I wouldn't need so much sleep."

Kathy yawned. "Your trouble, honey, is that you got used to the soft life."

"Maybe, but those bags under your eyes aren't just makeup, you know."

"I . . . know." Kathy yawned again. "Maybe if we could sleep when she does—"

"Su . . . re." Kathy had me yawning, too. Or at least something did. And Charity was lying there smiling, unaffected by the indecent hour. "Isn't there something you can give her?" I asked bluntly. "There are some big football games tomorrow, and I don't want to sleep through them."

"Blaine!"

"Well, we've got to do something! We really do need our sleep."

"You could always give her a blessing. She seems to understand them."

"Kath—"

"All right, O ye of little faith."

Although at first I was dubious, desperation forced me to agree. In my prayer I simply explained to Charity that we were getting older, and it would be very helpful if she would sleep at night and remain awake with us during the day. That was all, and it didn't seem to do any good. After the blessing she didn't get sleepy until long after daylight.

However, the next night she slept all night, and after that, except for when she was ill or in pain, she never again got her days and nights mixed up. In fact, the change was so dramatic that we began joking about the fact that we had discovered the sleep-all-night-through-blessings technique just six babies too late. What we never joked about, however, was our little angel daughter's amazing obedience.

We Hear from the Birth Family

In the months that followed, our thoughts went often to Charity's birth family. At the time, we did not know these people, yet in quiet moments Kathy and I often discussed them, wondering what they were like and if they were being comforted by the prayers of gratitude we so frequently offered up in their behalf. How thankful we were that the mother had chosen life for her unborn child. Not only would an abortion have denied Charity the right to experience a little mortality, but it would have denied all of us the privilege of loving her and getting to know her incredible spirit. Yet it would be terrifically hard, we felt, for a family to allow their baby daughter and granddaughter to be born, only to give her up. To be the beneficiary of their loss seemed especially difficult to us.

Occasionally Sharon would come and take Charity to them for a few hours, and we were made comfortable with this by thinking of how we would feel if our situations were reversed. Then one day Sharon appeared at our door with letters to us from the birth parents and grandparents. They were such sweet letters of support for us, but it was easy to see the pain and sorrow these people felt in their loss. Charity's birth mother wrote: "I would just like to tell you how thankful I am for the love you give to our precious little girl. I hope she has given you as much happiness as she has given me. The day she was born was the happiest day of my life. I'm so thankful that I still have the opportunity to see her grow and change. I hope that it hasn't imposed on you in any way. I don't know you, but I have a feeling in my heart that you are kind, loving people who care for our precious little angel baby. Thank you for everything you've done. . . . I'll never forget her and all the joy she's given to me. I'll love her throughout eternity. *Love and thanks forever.*"

It was no wonder, we thought as we read these letters, that Charity was such a special soul.

A SECOND SURGERY

◆

"Blaine, she's getting head pressure again. I know she is."

I shook my head more in dismay than disagreement. It was snowing outside, there were already six inches on the ground, and the last thing I wanted to do was set out for the hospital in a snowstorm. Besides, it was just a couple of days until Christmas, we had a major extended family celebration planned, and I didn't want to go through the hassle of unplanning it. But those weren't the real problems, and I knew it.

"Look at her soft spot," Kathy continued defensively. "See how it's bulging? That isn't normal, and you know it."

"I wasn't disagreeing with you, Kath. I . . . I just don't want poor little Charity to go through this again. I mean, that shunt is supposed to work for years, most likely for the rest of her life. If it isn't working, it will mean another surgery, and I don't know if any of us can take that again!"

The trouble was that at only four months of age, Charity was really starting to struggle, and I was worried. I knew she was at the age when her missing brain was supposed to be taking over from the brain stem, and it seemed likely that this was a sign of her impending death—just as we had been told to expect. So that afternoon I called Dr. Walker.

"Well, Kath," I said after the call, "he says that she might be dying, all right. But it might also be that her shunt is blocked. That's what keeps happening to that little boy who was operated on when we were there last time."

"So what do we do?"

"Keep her comfortable as much as we can. If there are still problems, Dr. Walker wants to see us right after the holidays."

And there were problems! Twice in the week between Christmas and New Year's, Charity reached such levels of stress that she briefly stopped breathing. She whimpered and cried all the time, her little body was rigid and trembling, and she could hardly bear being touched. Unfortunately, neither could she bear being left alone.

On January 4, 1989, after the doctor had determined that Charity's shunt was completely blocked, a new shunt was surgically implanted—this time on the opposite side of her head and body from the first one. And once again we and our tragically ill little girl were delivered over to the caring and compassion of the personnel at PCMC.

Following the surgery, one of the nurses noticed that Charity seemed to be having seizures. Dr. Fan Tait, a neurologist, was called in, and she felt an EEG was in order. The EEG was administered on the 7th, and the next morning we were invited to meet with Dr. Tait.

Spreading the EEG out on the table, Dr. Tait pointed out the electrical "spikes" Charity was experiencing. "This little girl's life is in danger," she said in a soft southern accent, her voice filled with genuine concern. "I believe we need to do something fast." Then she explained that individuals prone to seizures might spike every five minutes or so, which was considered serious. Charity's brain stem, on the other hand, was spiking as often as once every second or two, a situation Dr. Tait feared would destroy what limited brain tissue she had. Dr. Tait suggested phenobarbital to control the spiking, and we consented.

That afternoon as we sat with our innocent little girl, watching her tiny body twitch and suffer from the pain of the surgery and everything else she seemed forced to endure, I finally broke down. "It isn't fair," I said, burying my face in my hands. "Why should an innocent little baby like her be forced to suffer? Why does God allow it? If she's going to die anyway, why doesn't he just take her and stop all this craziness?"

"I . . . don't know," Kathy responded as tears fell from her eyes.

"I mean, how can a God of love allow this? She hasn't sinned; she'll never even be capable of sinning. If she's going to return automatically to God's presence, which I believe with all my heart, then what possible reason can there be for her to suffer like this?"

Instead of answering, for she had no answer, Kathy simply reached over and took my hand. If we couldn't understand, and if we couldn't comfort our forlorn little daughter, perhaps we could at least comfort each other.

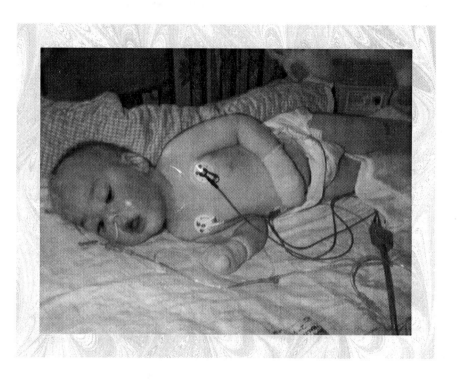

Charity after one of her shunt surgeries.

A Major Miracle

We brought Charity home on January 9, 1989, and again we were hopeful that we would not need to see the inside of PCMC again. After all, with both surgeries we had spent a total of nine days there, and we thought that surely Charity would now begin acting the way the medical experts had told us she should act—no health problems except for congestive things that would ultimately lead to death by pneumonia.

Unfortunately, again both we and they were wrong. Over the next few days Charity seemed to grow more and more ill. We didn't know what was wrong, the doctors didn't know what was wrong, and, if Charity knew, she couldn't tell us. All she could do was suffer, and we suffered helplessly with her.

And then one night—Friday the 13th of January, it happened to be—a miracle happened. All day Charity had grown worse. She was rigid and screaming, and we could do nothing that brought her any comfort. Twice Travis and I blessed her to be at peace. After the second blessing, when nothing had changed, Travis picked up some object and threw it against the wall.

"What's wrong with God?" he raged as tears of love and sympathy streamed down his cheeks. "Doesn't he see how much she's suffering? She hasn't done anything wrong! Why doesn't he stop this?"

Weeping with him, for Charity was truly suffering, neither Kathy nor I could offer an answer. We didn't understand it ourselves, so how could we explain it to our son?

"I . . . I'm sorry," Travis said a few moments later. "I know God doesn't cause this stuff. I just wish she didn't have to hurt so much."

"So do we," Kathy declared as she embraced him. "So do we!"

Throughout the day, as Charity continued to scream and tremble with pain, we prayed, singly and together, for some sort of relief. We even pleaded that, if it were possible, she would be allowed to pass away.

Calls to our pediatrician and PCMC brought no ideas on what might be wrong or what we could do, and even a visit to the local emergency room for tests failed to turn up a solution. Finally, sometime after midnight, as she exhaustedly rocked Charity back and forth, Kathy suddenly stopped. "I think I know what to do," she whispered. "Pour some warm water in the tub."

"Kath, it's nearly one in the morning. It isn't exactly the hour for bathing."

"It isn't a bath, hon. I have a feeling it will help her."

Quickly I ran a couple of inches of warm water into the bottom of the tub. Then, because Kathy's back problems were growing worse through the strain of holding Charity's rigid and arching little body so many hours each day, I took our baby and laid her in the water, her head supported in my hand.

For a few seconds she continued to scream. Then, abruptly, she stopped and looked directly at Kathy and me as though she could see us clearly. For three or four minutes she lay without moving a muscle. And then, to our everlasting surprise, she began kicking both legs at once (she had never been able to do that) and splashing her hands and feet in the water.

Then, to our further surprise, she smiled. Only briefly. But she smiled! Then came more splashing, more and bigger smiles, and suddenly, without any warning, she rolled her head back on my arm, her huge smile still there, and began to *giggle*.

We had never seen Charity laugh or do anything even remotely close to it. But for the next little while, as she splashed about in the tub, she giggled again and again. She would splash, roll her head to look at us, and giggle; splash, roll her head to look at us again, and giggle some more. It was the sweetest thing I had ever seen in my life, and as Kathy and I knelt beside her, breathing prayers of gratitude, plenty of tears joined the bathwater being joyfully splashed about by our daughter.

After perhaps twenty minutes, the giggling and even the smiling ceased, and she was back to kicking with just one leg at a time. We knew that our miracle of Charity being allowed to play in the tub just like all our other children had done was over. We dressed her and laid her in her crib, and in just moments she drifted into a sound sleep that lasted until late the next morning. Upon awakening, she seemed to be feeling much better.

Nearly three weeks later, following many additional examinations and tests, I wrote in a letter to our two children living overseas: "At least part of Charity's problems, it turns out, are because she is allergic to the phenobarbital. As for her laughter in the tub, no matter what we do that delightful behavior has not repeated itself. She still smiles occasionally and maybe kicks one leg, but there is no laughter or giggling, and the doctors, when we told them of the incident, told us there won't be (never could be, for that matter) because she lacks the brain capacity to express that sort of complex emotion.

"Yet we saw it clearly, which can mean only one thing—with the help of God this tiny child can be granted the capability of performing any activity or function any other child can perform."

Little did I know.

A Letter from Kathy

One night in February, I came upon Kathy weeping quietly on her knees. She told me that she had called a doctor with a question, and he, frustrated because Charity did not seem to follow "normal medical rules," had told her quite sharply than he had no more answers than she did—the implication being not to bother him anymore, that we were on our own.

"Heavenly Father is all I have left to turn to," she whispered. "And . . . and you." And then, as we held each other, she broke down and sobbed out her loneliness and grief.

"But I'll tell you what I'm going to do," she suddenly declared, swiping at her eyes. "I'm going to learn everything I can about Charity's problem, and I won't stop until I understand her. Then at least somebody will!"

The next day she went to work, studying everything she could get her hands on and grilling every doctor she could talk to with questions so detailed and sometimes so repetitive that I grew embarrassed. Still she kept after them until I was amazed at what she had learned.

One of the most interesting things she pursued was that Charity's condition was most commonly a manifestation of a disease called fetal alcohol syndrome. Of course, both of us understood that it wasn't possible to know exactly what had caused *our* daughter's probable stroke and subsequent hydranencephaly; the necessary tests, interviews, and evaluations had never been done. Generally speaking, however, diminished brain capacity, to one degree or another, is the second most common manifestation of fetal alcohol syndrome.

"So, alcohol abuse by the mother—" I started to question.

Kathy stopped me. "Not necessarily by the mother, Blaine, and not necessarily alcohol abuse, either. From what I read, extensive testing has shown that consumption of alcohol or drugs by either parent can cause fetal alcohol syndrome. And sometimes as little as one or two drinks or a single instance of drug abuse is enough to do the damage.

"Of course, the risk is greater if the mother uses these substances. And the more she uses them, the greater is the chance of damage to her fetus."

"And this may be what happened to Charity?"

Kathy shook her head. "We'll never know that. Remember, Charity's likely intrauterine stroke occurred early in the first trimester of her life. Charity's birth mother probably didn't even know she was pregnant at the time. She might simply have taken a painkiller for a bad headache, or perhaps she had a cold and took antihistamines or an alcohol-based cold remedy. That's why pregnant women are warned not to take medications from the moment they even think they might be expecting. Such drugs, or many other things that were out of the control of the birth parents, could have caused Charity's hydranencephaly."

I looked over some notes Kathy had taken:

A baby who has fetal alcohol syndrome will exhibit some or all of the following symptoms:
*Lower than average birth weight
*Small or nonexistent brain
*Lower-than-average intelligence

*Facial abnormalities, including a cleft lip and cleft palate, small eyes, and a small jaw
  *Heart defects
  *Abnormal arm and leg development
  *Poor sucking reflex
  *Irritability
  *Short stature
  *Difficulty sleeping
About one-fifth of babies with fetal alcohol syndrome die during the first few weeks after birth. Many of those who survive are physically and mentally disabled.

Besides a vast amount of knowledge such as this, Kathy also developed wonderful nursing skills as she spent hour after hour caring for Charity. Never had I imagined that someone could so completely devote her life to another. But, as with all things mortal, there was a price.

Though we could discover no medical reason for it, Kathy's back continued to deteriorate. Yet not once, under any condition, did she allow her own pain to slow her down. She was absolutely tenacious in her twenty-four-hour-a-day service to our little girl, and I will never in this life have words sufficient to express my love and admiration for what she did.

Through the winter and into the spring, Charity struggled with her reaction to phenobarbital. It took several hospitalizations and seemingly countless tests to finally discover a seizure medication she could tolerate. Meanwhile, our home life was in chaos. The people we were renting from were trying to sell their home and had asked us to show it for them, which we were happy (?) to do. My writing career was behaving more like a broken yo-yo than a rising star. To make economic matters worse, a Medicaid caseworker was threatening to cut off

Charity's desperately needed, and officially promised, Medicaid bene-
fits. And there were also the normal challenges of keeping up with four
kids in high school and junior high with all their activities, which
Kathy especially tried to be a part of. Besides my normal work, I did
most of the letter writing to our two children in Europe, and I spent a
lot of time telling them about the new little sister they had never yet
seen.

Through it all, I watched as two whom I had begun to think of as
heaven's daughters—Charity and my dear Kathy—faced each new crisis
and challenge with courage. And on the good days—the days at home
when all the two of them had to deal with were huge patches of
eczema, seizures, allergic reactions such as diarrhea and nausea, and
all the needs of a normal small baby—on these days, our home rang
with laughter and joy. Somehow Charity brought that happiness out
in all of us, no matter what she happened to be experiencing at the
moment.

Jane Adamson, a close family friend, wrote: "Charity had a way of
loving and of being able to communicate that was like no one else I
have ever known. I remember one experience very vividly. Kathy and I
had been standing next to Charity's bed, and Kathy had just finished
swabbing Charity's mouth and lips with water. She then left the room
to get something, leaving me with my hand on Charity's little hand. As
Kathy's voice got farther away, I felt Charity's body tense up, and I
could tell she was becoming frightened or nervous.

"I started to talk to her and tell her how much I loved her. I don't
remember all I said, but suddenly I was overcome with the strongest
feeling that Charity wanted me to tell her mother how much she loved
her, and how grateful she was for all that Kathy did to take care of her
every need. When Kathy came back into the room, I expressed these

thoughts to her, and instantly we both started to cry. A few minutes later I bent down and kissed Charity's soft little cheeks, and she looked at me and smiled the biggest smile, telling me as only she could, 'Thank you for giving Mommy my love.' It was so amazing how she could communicate."

Early that spring Kathy wrote our two absent children: "Since you have never met Charity, let me describe her for you. She now weighs fifteen pounds, so in spite of what the doctors expected, she is growing normally. Her hair had quite a bit of red in it initially, but now that it has all been shaved off it is coming in a darker brown with no red at all. Yet her eyebrows have a great deal of red in them, so maybe she will have auburn hair. It is still rather thin and short, but on the lower back of her head, left side, is a lovely lock of hair that is probably an inch and a half long—a token apparently left by the surgeons to appease my motherly instincts.

"Charity's skin is the color of pure porcelain, and her eyes are very unusual. When she feels good, her pupils expand until it seems her eyes are completely black. But when her head develops pressure, the pupils contract, and then she has the prettiest blue eyes one can imagine. There is a dark outer edge, then lighter blue, then occasionally a very thin line of darker blue before the black of the pupil. These gorgeous eyes that I love to gaze into are framed by long, dark, curly eyelashes that any girl would die for. They are very striking.

"Her left nostril is a little misshapen in what is the cutest little button nose. She has what one of my friends calls an 'Arby hat' mouth, very dainty and petite. Her cheeks are chubby (she reminds me so much of Tami and Michelle as babies that I can't imagine we actually adopted her), and her ears are set close against her head and are so cute. Because of her hydranencephaly she holds her thumbs in all the

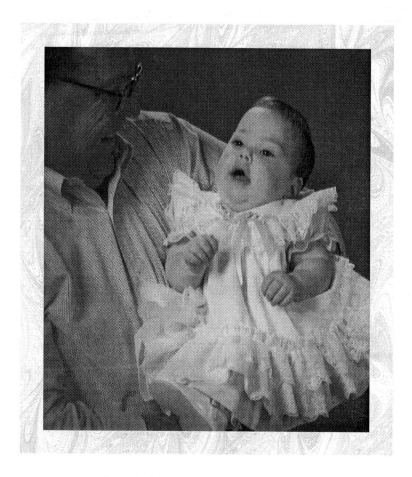

Blaine holding nine-month-old Charity.

time, with her fingers usually clenched over them. She stiffens her arms and legs and curls her toes straight down when she is frightened or in pain, and it is very difficult to bend her arms and legs unless she is perfectly relaxed.

"She rarely cries just to hear herself, but she has a good, loud cry when she wants to let it out. But what really breaks my heart is the pathetic little rapid sobs she makes when she is in pain. Some of the doctors still don't believe she is capable of pain, but I know very well they are wrong. This child really suffers from pain, and in the moments when she is free of it, her beautiful smile declares her joy to all the world. She also talks occasionally—sweet little baby sounds that I love to hear. But our family's favorite sound is Charity's snort, which is very loud and occurs every time she sighs or takes a deep breath—not infrequently. We have no idea why she does this, but we absolutely love it!

"She is a very patient baby, often lying in bed for an hour or more after awakening, without any complaint. And that, by the way, is the only time we can get her to smile. In the morning, when she is well-rested, if we go in and call her name very quietly, she will give the sweetest smile in the whole world. She responds to us at other times by kicking or using her eyes, but our favorite responses are her smiles.

"Of course, her doctors don't believe she is really smiling, but they haven't seen it. One of these days Charity will show them, and they will know.

"There are other things she does that we were told she would never do: she knows her name, recognizes our voices, and responds to each of us differently. It is so interesting to see. Nate is reserved with her, and so she is reserved with him. Travis isn't so much reserved as he is shy around her. He is nevertheless quite protective of her, and nuzzles her neck with his nose when he thinks he isn't being watched. Charity saves her sweetest smiles for him. Dan and Michelle she loves to play and dance with, and she gets all excited whenever they speak to her. She really loves them, and they know it.

"I have never seen Blaine so in love with a child, and Charity loves him just as much. She especially enjoys all the cute little love songs he makes up for her. They make her absolutely beam! More and more I need his help, so he is now getting up at 4:00 in the morning to do his writing. He says it isn't a problem, but I can tell how tired he is.

"And me? Well, I'm just Mom. I'm the one who has to worry about all the little things like swabbing her mouth to keep it moist, getting her the medications on time, feeding her, keeping her warm (it seems easy for her to get cold), and of course bathing, dressing, and changing her, and doing everything I can think of to make her comfortable. A good share of my day is spent trying to make her more comfortable so she will relax. In fact, I spend hours and hours each day holding and rocking her—and constantly the Holy Spirit whispers, 'Cherish these moments.' Charity puts up with all of my fiddling with her body, but sometimes I can tell that she really grows tired of it. Yet I can feel her love for me, too, and it is the most wonderful feeling in the world. Her love makes all of the hard times worthwhile."

A Thought-Provoking Musing

***

"You know, honey," Kathy said one day when I came in to spell her with Charity's bottle, "somehow this little girl can think, and I have proof of it."

Reaching down, I lifted Charity and began nuzzling her. "I believe you, hon. But proof?"

"Well, it's proof to me. She knows the single pacifier she likes and always rejects the others. She knows exactly which brand of formula she likes and refuses anything else. She lies flat without complaint, but she protests loudly at both her swing and her baby seat. On the other hand, if the children or us swing her or hold her upright in our arms, she doesn't protest at all, but seems to enjoy it. To me, these are proofs."

I nodded.

"Charity is anything but a vegetable," Kathy concluded, "and I can't imagine how any thinking person—especially medical people who have been trained to reason—could be deceived into such an idiotic conclusion as so many of them seem to have come to."

As Charity lay in my arms contentedly working her bottle, her fathomless eyes locked on my own, I had to agree. There was definitely an intelligence there, an intelligence that had nothing to do with the human organ called a brain.

When Tami returned from England near the end of February, we learned again how obedient Charity was and how her amazing "mind" operated. Of course, Charity was not used to Tami's voice, and each time Tami held her she began to cry. After three days of this, I finally took Charity (again at Kathy's suggestion) and went alone into the living room, where I explained in a blessing who Tami was and how badly she was feeling about Charity's tears.

Charity never again cried in Tami's arms. In fact, the two of them became extremely close, and each learned how to help and love the other. Later Tami wrote: "I'm not sure how to say how I feel about Charity, and how grateful I am that she has been in my life. The words 'I love her' seem so inadequate. Nothing I might ever say could express the depth of my feelings. Every memory of her I treasure. I look forward to the day when we can embrace and talk face to face, and I can hear her words as well as feel her incredibly beautiful spirit."

Having learned my lesson, when Steve came home from Norway a couple of months later, I immediately gave Charity a blessing of introduction, and without hesitation she welcomed Steve wholeheartedly into her life. "My experiences with Charity and my feelings for her," Steve writes, "have filled me with wonder and profound love. Charity couldn't do much physically, but I have never seen anyone change the lives of so many people for the better. She is a remarkably obedient person."

And Travis, who had only recently traveled to South America, wrote: "I love Charity tons—she's just an angel. Go ahead. Tell me that sounds strange. But no matter what it sounds like, it is the honest-to-gosh truth. I love partaking of the Spirit that she seems to constantly possess. I love that kid to death, and I find myself thinking of her all the time."

We were so struck by Charity's ability to receive communication and understanding through blessings that, from then on, we used blessings to inform her of whatever was happening in our family. For instance, if for any reason Kathy and I were given a brief break together, I first blessed Charity to know that we were leaving only temporarily. She was then peaceful for her tenderhearted caregivers. On the rare occasions when I forgot to do this, however, Charity was brokenhearted by our absence, and showed it through her tears.

On April 6, 1989, we all gathered in court, where a judge granted our petition and Charity Afton legally became our daughter. Even the birth certificate filed with the state reflects Kathy and me as her parents. Then, in a sweet religious ceremony on May 26, 1989, Charity was made a spiritual part of our family. Afterward, as we visited, the elderly man who had performed the ceremony made a remark that burned like fire into my thinking, and that I will not forget as long as I live. "In our church we believe in the ministering of angels," he said as he held Kathy's and my hands from his wheelchair. "It would be interesting to know why you and your family have been selected to minister *to* one."

Well, we didn't know. But with this man's witness, we knew with absolute surety that Charity was indeed an angel—a powerful being of pure sweetness and light who had honored and blessed us with her presence in ways we would never in mortality fully understand.

What mattered that others did not understand or even denied such intangible, spiritual things? What mattered that at times her care seemed hard? What mattered the loss of a little personal freedom, the spending of a few extra dollars, or even hundreds of nights' sleep given up in her service? To have the privilege of dwelling even briefly with one of God's holy angels was worth any price we had to pay.

REACHING OUT

Despite such lofty ideals, life was difficult. On top of Charity's suffering and the strain of Kathy's unending sacrifice in her behalf, even day-to-day things seemed to be getting harder. Forced to move again by the sale of the home we had been renting, it seemed to me that my mind—and my life—were always in chaos. I could never find the books and other research materials I felt I needed for my writing (at one point, too tired to think of moving my collection of research books one more time, I had simply given thirty-nine boxes of them away), and I could not seem to focus on the work I was supposed to be doing. In fact, as I sat at my computer one morning in late August, it occurred to me that in three months I had not completed even one entire chapter in the manuscript I had promised to submit to my publisher the previous spring. For a man who carried the responsibility of recovering financially and supporting his family's needs, it was hard not to think of myself as a failure. To others I did a lot of joking about being a wanderer and a vagabond upon the earth, but in my heart I knew it was no laughing matter.

Worse, although many family members and friends had expressed sweet support for our decision to adopt Charity, and were helping however they could, there were a few, some even within our own family, who were very critical. One chose to avoid much association with

Charity because she was not of "our bloodline"; another regularly crit-icized us for giving too much of our time to what he termed a "brain-dead" baby; others continually dropped unsubtle hints regarding our amazing foolishness for having adopted her in the first place. On three separate occasions I was angrily denounced for what I was "forcing" Kathy to endure. The kids picked up on some of this at school, which both confused and hurt them, and one of my brothers, attending a local ball game one night, listened as some "friends" of ours seated next to him (who did not know him) made jokes about our stupidity. It was all he could do to restrain himself from "letting them have it," as he put it later.

I did my best to shield Kathy from this nonsense, but what she did encounter hurt her deeply, and it had a noticeable effect upon me. Isn't it strange how we can let the opinions of the few affect us more than those of the many? In fact, there were days when I found myself won-dering the same things our critics had voiced, and when no matter how hard I prayed, I couldn't seem to find any comfort. Looking back, I can see that I was falling apart as rapidly as were Kathy and Charity. I was just doing it in a different direction.

Thank the Lord we had little Charity in our lives. Her smile could salve even the worst of my wounds, and many were the times when, as I held her and tried to comfort her in her pain, she ended up comfort-ing me. I am not able to describe the soothing effect she had upon my soul, neither will I ever be able to sufficiently thank God for the great blessing she became to us. What I can do is state that, though I didn't understand her pain, I came to know absolutely that our adopting her had been no mistake, no foolishness, no stupidity. She was where God wanted her to be, and it became increasingly obvious to me, as that summer passed, that the blessing was far more ours than it ever could be hers.

I don't mean to give the impression that our family's life, after Charity's arrival, was one continual round of crisis and pain. It wasn't. In spite of her serious health problems, Charity had a remarkable number of good days during her first year of life, and on those days we were a pretty normal bunch. There was a lot of laughter and goofing off in our home, probably too much teasing (it usually became unkind), and all sorts of regular chores and projects. The children were involved in both school and extracurricular activities. As they got old enough, they all held part-time jobs, and our girls loved singing and drama, while local and national sports were of prime importance to our four sons.

In addition, Kathy and I did our best to see that we were all involved in family things—trips to nearby places of interest, games, puzzles, video movies, regular family discussions about religion and sundry other topics, church activities, and so forth. We also refereed arguments, tried to stop out-and-out battles, insisted on homework being done before ten million other "more important" things, and even managed occasionally to get a night out alone with each other.

Mostly, though, after our tiny daughter's arrival in our home, we became a family of unabashed Charity watchers. She was like a sweet magnet drawing us all to her, and none of us could get enough of holding her, dancing with her, singing to her, and simply being with her.

"That little girl touches me in ways I have never been touched," I told Kathy one day. "I absolutely love and adore her. But I am also in awe of her; I cry with joy when she smiles at me; I can hardly keep myself from smothering her with hugs and kisses; I find myself constantly singing to her; I feel guilty when I am around her because I don't know how to care for her the way you do, and yet I know with every fiber of my being that she loves me unconditionally; and I don't think I will ever in this life stop wondering who she really is. Yet if I were asked what Charity does to affect me like that, I don't know if I could give a sensible answer."

"Sure you could," Kathy responded. "She may never talk or sing or run or jump or play like other little girls, which are the things we always talk about when we describe our children, but she does do something. She radiates. She is like a lamp with a bulb that seems to grow brighter the older she gets, radiating love and joy and peace to any who come near and want to feel it."

Kathy was right. I have come to believe that the brain is important only because it provides the physical house for that part of the eternal spirit called the mind. Charity's mind was a real part of her spirit, and brilliant. Despite the fact that she didn't have a brain to work with, she was continually radiating or communicating love and gratitude in a way no one else I have ever known could do it. Practically everyone who ever came near her felt this and was changed by it.

The older Charity grew, the more frightening, complicated, and time-consuming her care became, and she quickly passed the stage where we could ask a local teenager to come and sit with her. To their everlasting credit, a few precious women overcame their fears and came to us, offering their time, service, and love when we needed to get away, even for just an hour or two. Truthfully, I don't know what we would have done without their help.

LaDawn Godwin, one of these great women, says: "I treasure every minute I was able to spend with Charity. Sometimes she and I would just laugh together, and I thought how amazing it was to see the things that struck her as funny. I would be having trouble with her formula, or I would be combing her hair and run into a snarl, or maybe trying to bathe her and drop the soap or something else just as silly, and all of a sudden Charity's little body would begin shaking and she would start to laugh. That would make me laugh, and then we would giggle together like two young girls. I truly feel that we had a special bond, not like a baby-sitter or substitute mother so much as like best friends or maybe sisters."

"There were several times when we as a family had the privilege of having Charity in our home for two or three days," Rita Nelson, another of Charity's caregivers, adds. "Each of us loved going into her room to visit with her and to feel of her spirit—that is the way we communicated with this little girl, spirit to spirit. Charity always inspired in us a greater appreciation for each other and for life."

Sharon Lambert, who also helped us with our daughter, concludes: "Each Sunday I looked forward to my short visit with Charity, whom I always called 'Little Lamb' because of her amazing, porcelain-like complexion. There was such a sweet, calm feeling of peace and serenity in her room. Holding her and rocking her gave me time to meditate and reflect upon my direction in life. She inspired me to want to be my best self, and to try harder to reach out to others. A few times Richard and I also had the privilege of having her in our home. This was such a blessing, because her presence of love and peace was felt by our children and grandchildren. Charity had her own way of singing and laughing and spreading joy, and we were blessed to enjoy some of those times with her.

"I'm certain Charity knows now what strength and courage, friendship and love she gave so freely to me and my family. She changed our lives forever, and I thank her for that."

Praying for Death

🌿 "Honey, I'm scared for her. I don't think she can take a lot more."

"I don't either," I said as I held Kathy's hand. "I couldn't, I know that!"

It was the end of August, 1989, and we were back at PCMC sitting in the waiting room as Dr. Linda Book ran tests concerning reflux problems Charity had apparently developed. It was amazing how many different kinds of problems our little angel had developed, especially since none of them had anything to do with respiration. In fact, she had never come down with any of the normal childhood illnesses, not even a cold. Once again she was not doing what the medical profession had expected.

However, she had been terribly ill during this hospitalization, so sick and in so much pain that she had lost her ability to suck. For her to obtain nourishment, an NG (nasal-gastric) tube had been inserted through her nostril and into her stomach, a tube that Kathy and I would have to replace weekly, and from then on for the rest of her life she took all her nourishment, liquids, and medications through those tubes.

Kathy says: "Changing Charity's NG tube was extremely difficult, and it took both Blaine and me to do it. First the old tube had to be removed. Because the tape holding it in place had been there all week, we had to remove it with special swabs so we wouldn't tear the skin or cause infection. Next, Blaine held her head and neck steady while I inserted into her other nostril the new tube, coated with lubricant. It was never easy getting it down her throat, past her lungs, and into her stomach. Not only were we worried about it injuring her or going into the wrong place, but every time, Charity gagged and coughed and tried to twist away from it. The nurses told us it was a very painful procedure, and Charity agreed. Sometimes when it took three or four tries because the tube kinked or whatever, Blaine and I wept to see her suffering. Needless to say, all three of us dreaded tube-changing day. And all of us breathed a sigh of relief once it was in and we had a whole week of peace ahead of us."*

Charity spent her first birthday in PCMC, and I was overwhelmed with the way the hospital personnel went out of their way to ensure that not only she, but Kathy and I as well, had a special day. All day long, nurses walked in singing happy birthday songs. Charity was given a beautiful little hand-sewn blanket that had been donated by someone for that very purpose. Balloons and a tiny cake with a single candle were brought in. Even Ronald McDonald came and posed with Charity for our camera. In spite of Charity's struggles, it truly was an enjoyable day—made so, I know, by the extra caring of our PCMC friends.

Many of our family members also made the trek to the hospital in order to celebrate with Charity, and it was easy for me to see that this challenged little angel had wormed her way as deeply into their hearts as she had into mine. One day Nate, twenty-two years old now, came in and stood beside her bed, silent tears streaming down his face. After he was gone, the mother of the other child in the room took Kathy's hand. "I don't think I've ever seen anything so beautiful," she said. "For

---

* A surgically implanted gastric (stomach) tube is available, which in some respects would have been a lot easier on all of us. But because every medical person we ever visited expected Charity's immediate demise, we were strongly encouraged not to put her through that additional surgery.

a boy that age to have the maturity to weep over his little sister is remarkable. I can tell your family really loves her." And she was right. We did.

"You know," Nate said as we walked down the hall together, "I thought you and Mom were crazy for adopting Charity. Since you did, I figured why go to all the trouble and endure the pain that would surely come about through emotional attachment. But she won't let me get away with it. Part of her mission here, I believe, is to teach love to all who come in contact with her, even on the most casual level. And that includes me. She is her name in its purest form, and I can feel her love, Dad. I . . . I hope it isn't too late for me to love her back."

In late September Charity was again hospitalized for more tests, which were inconclusive. By the latter part of October, however, it was becoming evident that the shunt was not functioning properly, though no one could be sure why. Tests run in early November indicated that the shunt was overdraining rather than the reverse.

"When you draw too much cerebrospinal fluid from Charity's cranial cavity," Dr. Walker explained, "it creates a situation much like a dry socket where a tooth has been extracted. And like a dry socket, the pain of too much fluid loss in the head is incredible. In other words, Charity is experiencing something like continuous massive migraine headaches."

"Can anything be done?" I asked.

"Well, we can try adjusting the shunt. If that doesn't work, then we'll replace it with a shunt with a higher pressure valve."

In sorrow Kathy and I gazed down at our little daughter, who had finally grown her hair back out. Now, I thought, she was going to have it shaved off once again.

"With pain like that," Kathy said as she focused on the most important thing, "it's no wonder she's been so miserable and uncomfortable. She whimpers and quakes and trembles constantly. Can we do this soon, doctor?"

"Of course. We'll adjust the shunt right away, and then we'll give her a couple of weeks to see how she's getting along."

And so with heavy hearts Kathy and I prepared ourselves to watch our suffering little daughter endure another shunt surgery.

To help Charity's overdrainage we kept her head lowered, and Dr. Walker performed the shunt adjustment in the middle of November. When that was not successful, Charity was hospitalized again, and on December 5 her shunt was removed and another with a higher pressure valve was inserted on the other side.

Taking our suffering little angel home, we set about trying to get Christmas organized and a little shopping done. But Charity was not doing well at all, and with each passing day, it became more evident that her condition was deteriorating. She spent less time sleeping—consequently, so did we—and her poor little body was constantly racked with pain.

On December 19, we were forced to admit our little daughter to PCMC again. There Dr. Walker determined that her newest shunt had malfunctioned, and upon his recommendation we prepared ourselves and our children at home for another ordeal of surgery. To Kathy and me, this meant the sorrow of watching one child suffer while older ones at home were neglected. To the children at home, it meant not only that we would be gone—sometimes day and night—until Charity was ready to be discharged, including over Christmas, but also that they might never again see their beloved little sister. It was truly a difficult time for us all.

The removal of the shunt from Charity's right side, as well as the placement of a new shunt on her left side, took place on December 22. But Charity had been so beaten up by all that had transpired already in her short life that she did not bounce quickly back. She simply lay in her crib that day and the next, whimpering but not crying, and tearing our hearts out with her almost silent suffering.

"Just look at her," I whispered to Kathy as she was wheeled past us and out the door for another CT scan on the 23rd. "How does the poor little thing keep going? And why? Why doesn't she just give up and die?"

"Have you prayed for that?" Kathy asked quietly.

"That she can die? Every day, sometimes dozens of times. I love being around her, Kath, but not at this price. I can't stand it! With all my heart I wish she could be taken so she can finally know peace."

"I've prayed for the same thing." Kathy rubbed her tired, red-rimmed eyes. "But I keep wondering. What if Heavenly Father doesn't want her to die?"

I sighed and leaned back in the chair. "I think of that, too. I guess you could say I pray out of both sides of my mouth, because even when I'm asking for her to go I'm also asking that if the Lord wills it, she be made well so she can stay. To tell you the truth, Kath, I don't know if I could stand having her leave us."

"I . . . don't, either," Kathy responded as she wiped some tears that were suddenly escaping. "So lately I've just been praying that you and I can have the strength to endure whatever Heavenly Father has planned."

"I think we're going to need it," I muttered.

"Do *you* think she's going to die?" Kathy pressed. "Soon, I mean?"

Well, I didn't know. But for some reason I didn't think so. At sixteen months of age, Charity wasn't a very big person. Yet despite all the horrors she had been forced to endure, she clung to life with a tenacity that amazed me.

"Not yet," I finally responded. "I don't think she's ready to go."

"Then we'd better pray for her endurance, too," Kathy responded as she took my hand. "The way it looks, she must surely know something that we don't know, some reason why she feels she must stay."

"But why? Why would God require such a thing of her? I'm telling you, Kath, I don't understand!"

It simply made no sense to me that an innocent little child would be required to suffer so deeply, so continually. Neither did I understand why she had been born without a brain in the first place. It wasn't the question of what had caused the intrauterine stroke that was bothering me, as much it was, Why her? Why this perfect little girl?

I didn't know, but it surely didn't seem fair. If people could just see what I had seen over the last sixteen months, I thought. If they could only feel what I had felt as I had watched an innocent, beloved child suffer and struggle through practically every day of her mortal life! If they could weep as I had wept while watching other little boys and girls toddling into their proud parents' arms or chasing a butterfly or petting a frisky puppy or uttering their first words and then forming them into sentences—if they could see those things and then know that their own little child would never experience such joys, such accomplishments—if they could know that they would never speak with their little girl or communicate verbally, then perhaps they would understand why I was having such a struggle.

A SUFFERING LITTLE CHILD

It was Sunday, the morning of Christmas Eve. Over the hospital intercom the joyous sounds of Christmas were playing, though the music—the Christmas songs I had loved my entire life—could not break through. Instead, the noise in the room with the suffering babies drowned it out. Besides their crying and whimpering, between the two infants there were one IVAC intravenous pump, one Kangaroo feeding tube pump, two cardiac monitors, an Oximeter, an Esophageal pH Probe monitor, and a Sleep Study machine, each beeping and humming and sounding what seemed like constant alarms to let the nurses know when problems were developing.

As the piercing alarm on Charity's cardiac monitor sounded for maybe the tenth time in thirty minutes, indicating that a lead wire had pulled loose again, I rose to my feet in desperation.

"This place," I muttered to my wife, "is driving me crazy!"

She looked at me sympathetically. "I can tell you're upset, but I don't think it's the hospital's fault."

"Maybe, maybe not." I stared out the window as a Life-Flight helicopter lifted noisily off its pad, another sign of the pain with which we were surrounded. Groaning inwardly, I turned back into the room. "No, it isn't the hospital. In fact, I feel very thankful for it and all these doctors and nurses. They're great, and I don't know what we'd ever do without them. It's just that . . . well, I can't take any more of this noise!"

"Don't you think it's because you're tired?" Kathy asked.

She had a point. After all, I had been up with Charity all night. "Maybe," I admitted, "but I'm still getting out of here."

"Where will you go?" Kathy asked, not trying to dissuade me. "It's Sunday morning."

"Yeah," I replied, "and tonight is Christmas Eve, so everything is closed. Maybe I'll just go wander the halls here in the hospital."

"The children in the other rooms are just as ill as our baby," she said gently, somehow understanding that it wasn't really the noise that was bothering me.

Slowly I nodded, while tears filled my eyes once again. "I . . . I just can't bear to see her suffer like this. All this pain just doesn't seem fair! If there were only something I could do!"

"Honey," Kathy chided softly, "we've done everything we can do, so we need to leave it to the Lord. Besides, you knew it would be like this when we agreed to bring her into our family. Don't you remember that we both promised, in prayer, that we wouldn't complain, no matter how bad things got?"

I remembered, but it still seemed so unfair. "Here it is Christmas," I said, "and while millions of children are happily anticipating tomorrow morning's toys, she's stuck here in the hospital without even the mental ability to understand what she's missing. What a lousy place to spend Christmas! What a lousy hand to be dealt in life!"

"You don't really feel like this," Kathy said softly as she put her hand on my arm. "I know you don't. I've heard you tell too many people how thankful you are for Charity."

Our daughter lay still, but every few seconds she would writhe with pain as she whimpered and cried out for relief. The whole scene wrenched my heart more than I could have imagined possible, and knowing that there was no real hope for her mortal future made the situation seem just that much worse.

Blinking back tears of despair, I finally left the room and made my way down the hall. The waiting room, I thought moments later as I sank into an empty couch, was at least a little more quiet, and the suffering patients were thankfully out of sight.

For once the TV was off, and other than the soft snoring of an elderly grandfather and the Christmas music playing softly over the intercom, the room was blissfully still.

Glancing around, I looked past the old and well-read magazines to an early edition of the Sunday paper that someone had left scattered on the floor. "Jerks!" I grumbled softly. "Where were they raised? In a barn?" For a moment I thought of gathering the paper and losing myself in it. Somehow, though, I didn't have the energy to even drag myself to it, let alone read. So I lay back, closed my eyes, and—and saw in my mind the terribly wounded form of my tiny daughter.

"No!" I breathed as I forced my eyes open again. "I don't want to see that. I can't bear to see it—"

Across the room stood a brightly decorated Christmas tree, a glowing angel perched on the uppermost needled spire. For a moment I studied her—I believe it was a "her"—noting her wings, the halo, the scepter in her hand. Everything about her looked rumpled, battered, crooked. The gold halo flopped down in front of her face, her scepter was bent, her wings were crooked, and I could see a rip in her dress.

"Looks like a kid decided to play with her," I muttered grimly, my heart filled with disgust. "Or maybe a dozen kids, the way she looks.

Good grief! With all the money they take in, you'd think the hospital could afford some decent Christmas ornaments! Cheapskates!"

Over the intercom someone was singing, *"Hark, the herald angels sing, glory to the newborn King."* Tearing my eyes from the tattered angel, I found myself thinking again of my little girl, her tiny body savaged by the medical procedures she had been forced to endure.

"Oh, man!" I thought as I closed my eyes against this vision. "How did I ever let myself get into such a mess? How did I let Kathy get into it? What are we doing here?

"Dear God," I found myself pleading, "please help me to understand—"

I was watching but not seeing the lonely, tattered angel on top of the Christmas tree when a group of carolers moved through the waiting room. Blinking to clear my mind, I glanced at the clock and discovered, to my surprise, that I had been sitting there more than an hour. With a heavy sigh I rose to my feet and headed back to Charity's room. Probably, I thought, Kathy would need a break.

"The First Noel" and "Silent Night" were the songs the carolers were singing as I made my way past them, songs celebrating the birth of Christ. But in my loneliness and sorrow the words bounced off me, making no impression.

"Honey," Kathy suggested as I came through the door, "why don't we both go downstairs to attend church?"

"I know we need a break, Kath. But what about little Charity? One of us should stay here with her."

"I'll take care of Charity," a young nurse said brightly as she came into the room and into our conversation. "As a Christmas present, of course. You two go ahead and go. You both look like you could use a break."

"What were you doing?" I grumbled teasingly. "Eavesdropping?"

She laughed, not sounding tired even though she had been on a constant run from crisis to crisis since 7:00 that morning. Quickly she shut off a piercing alarm and began readjusting the lead-in wires to our baby's chest. "Nurses have 20/20 hearing," she replied as she worked. "That's part of our training. Besides, I'd love to spend more time with your darling little girl. She just radiates Christmas cheer! Now hurry or you'll be late."

I smiled weakly and thanked her. Then together Kathy and I gave a longing look at our tiny daughter and departed for the bottom floor of the hospital, where church services were being held.

We had never attended the ecumenical Sunday service at the Medical Center before, and I watched with interest as people associated with the hospital took care of the program. One of the staff took charge, and the mother of a patient led the singing—all Christmas hymns that day. A sister of another patient played hymns on the piano, a young patient prayed, and two fathers of very ill babies and a young patient wearing an awkward-looking brace made some appropriate remarks regarding Christmas and the birth of Jesus Christ.

I watched all these people giving service, thought of the pain each of them was covering up but still feeling—pain I had never imagined existed until we had been granted our own challenged daughter—and suddenly I realized that I was weeping.

I should probably admit that I have a tendency to bawl at the drop of a hat, for which my kids persecute me endlessly. But somehow I sensed that this was different—very different. For one thing, I could not stop weeping. I could not even slow down. For another, my chest felt like it was burning with a wonderful sort of warmth, and suddenly I seemed to be completely filled with a sense of love.

"Are you all right?" Kathy whispered anxiously as she reached and took my hand.

I nodded, fumbling for my handkerchief. "I . . . I feel so strange, almost like I'm on fire or something."

"Are you sick?"

"No! Not at all. In fact, it's the most wonderful feeling I've ever had. I feel like I want to hug people—everybody! Can you imagine me doing that? I want to tell them how much I love them; how much God loves them. . . . Kath, do you think maybe the Lord is giving me the understanding I prayed for earlier?"

"I don't know, but wouldn't it be wonderful if he was?"

Scant moments later my wife wiped at her own eyes and squeezed my hand. "I . . . I'm feeling it, too," she whispered. "This is so amazing! I'm sure this is an answer to our prayers."

As the service continued, we noticed that others in the congregtion seemed to be feeling the same sweet, peaceful spirit, for they were responding much as we were. After the service we overheard one or two quiet remarks of confirmation, and as we returned to the fourth floor, Kathy and I wonderingly discussed our experience. The intense spiritual feeling had lasted for several minutes, perhaps twenty or thirty, and then, just as suddenly as it had come, it had gone again. We marveled at that, marveled that we should have been allowed to share it with each other, and, alone once again with our suffering little Charity, we gave silent thanks that the Lord had allowed the power of his Spirit to bring the comfort so many of us had no doubt been praying for.

Now, I thought, if I could just make certain that my daughter also knew—

THE DISHWASHER

◆

Early that afternoon I sat alone in the cafeteria. Kathy had eaten first and I had followed, eating separately so that one of us could remain with Charity. As I took my first bite, I noticed a young man watching me. He was an employee–a dishwasher, I thought–and I knew that he was mentally challenged.

"Oh, no," I thought as I saw his sober gaze resting on me, "I hope he doesn't want to sit with me. I don't feel like making conversation with someone like him–not today. There is so much that I want to think about, to ponder."

I watched furtively and was relieved when he finally sat at the next table. Slowly I continued to eat, but I could tell that he wasn't eating. In fact, even without looking I knew that he was simply waiting, watching me. He hadn't touched his food.

"Come on," I grumbled at him in my mind, "just eat your dinner. Can't you tell that I want to be left alone?"

Still the young man said nothing; he just watched me. So I took another bite, and as I did so, from out in the hall came the sounds of another group of Christmas carolers–"*I heard the bells on Christmas day/Their old familiar carols play,/And wild and sweet the words repeat/Of peace on earth, good will to men.*

As I listened to the song, from out of nowhere something inside me spoke—a voice that I recognized immediately as my own occasionally hyperactive conscience.

"What's the matter with you?" I was asked rather abruptly. "Don't you believe in Christmas?"

"Sure I do," I thought in surprise.

"Then why don't you act like it?" the inner voice questioned. "You enjoyed a marvelous spiritual experience this morning, wherein the Lord spoke great peace to your soul. Where is your *good will to men* that you cannot reach out and speak peace to the soul of another?"

"I . . . uh . . ."

"Did you think that the Holy Spirit came only to bless and comfort you?" the voice persisted. "Or the physically ill? Did you think that, outside of the little children who are patients here, you and your wife were the only ones who felt it? You know very well that Jesus suffered in order that he might bring peace and comfort to all his children, no matter what their age or why they are suffering. Like the little angel on the tree upstairs, they are also tattered. But Christ loves them more for that, not less, and they remain his angels still."

"I . . . I hadn't thought of it quite like that . . ." I stammered to myself as I saw in my mind the angel on the Christmas tree upstairs, the angel who had been so abused and battered by others, the angel *I* had been so critical of.

Suddenly my mind was filled with images of the children in the hospital, the ones I had seen that very morning. In one room a child who was battling leukemia had been playing a game with his mother. He was hairless, but he was also smiling, so at least the nausea from his chemotherapy was gone. Two rooms I had passed were isolation rooms where the children were suffering with RSV, respiratory syncytial virus, which led to bronchiolitis. Highly infectious, these isolated children seemed to be in a great deal of pain. In another room lay a tiny girl who had been born with ventricular septal defect, a hole between the lower chambers of her heart. She had also been born without corneas in her eyes, and there had been much urgency as the staff tried to ready her heart so she could have the strength to undergo cornea transplants. I had also seen children who suffered from gastroenteritis and meningitis and various traumas caused by accidents of one sort or another. In fact, I had been told that one entire unit in the hospital was the multiple trauma unit, where children with multiple organ injuries from accidents, abuse, and so forth, were cared for.

Indeed they *were* tattered angels, every single one of them! And every one of them was loved of Christ.

"You need to think of them," I told myself. "And you need to repent while you're at it. After all, this *is* Christmas. If God the Father and his Beloved Son could send forth their Holy Spirit on a Christmas visit to all these children, and if seeing pain in these innocent ones is as distressing to you as you have been claiming, then couldn't you perhaps give a little time and love to one who must suffer much longer than your Charity will ever need to suffer—a little *peace on earth, good will to men?*"

Instantly I was encompassed with great guilt. And slowly I nodded my head.

"Besides, my friend," the voice of my conscience continued, now gentle again. "you have always loved Christmas. Here is a chance to make this one just a little bit better than any you have ever enjoyed."

Feeling terrible, I solemnly apologized to heaven for my arrogance. Then, with the beginnings of a genuine smile on my countenance, I turned to meet the gaze of one tattered angel, one of God's truly elect

on the earth, whose friendship and Christlike love I would soon come
to appreciate.

"Are you alone?" he asked the instant my eyes met his. His face was
gravely serious.

Slowly I nodded.

"Can I eat with you?"

I suppose I still hesitated briefly. But then I nodded again and
agreed. Quickly he stood, picked up his tray, and stepped to my table.

"My name's Fred," he told me as he carefully arranged his tray and
sat down. "What's your name?"

I told him.

"That's a good name," he said sincerely. "I have a warm spirit. Want
to feel it?"

Surprised, I wondered how to respond. After all, I knew that this
young man was mentally deficient, at least to some extent. But he was
also very polite, and though he had not smiled even once, which
seemed a little strange, my inclination was to treat him as I would treat
any other adult.

"You say you have a warm spirit?" I asked, trying to be as polite as
he seemed to be.

"Uh-huh. Want to feel it?"

"Sure," I replied, doing my best not to grin. "But how do you—"

Before I could finish my question, Fred reached out and, with quite
a bit of force, clapped his hand on my head just above my forehead.

"See how warm my hand is?" he asked matter-of-factly. "That's
because of my warm spirit."

For a moment I sat in startled silence, almost stunned by the
incredible warmth of Fred's hand. It *was* warm, almost hot, but it was

definitely not unpleasant. For a moment I wondered how my own hand would feel.

"Do you have a warm spirit?" he asked as he suddenly pulled his hand away, almost as if he were reading my mind.

"I . . . I don't know."

"Here," he said, reaching out and taking my hand in his. "Put it on my head and let me feel."

I let my hand be guided to his head. He held it still for a few seconds, and then gently he took it away. "It's a little warm," he declared as he took his first bite of food. "Not as warm as mine, though. Do you know why mine is so warm?"

Dumbly I shook my head.

"Because I love people," he said simply. "Love is what makes my spirit warm."

"How . . . do you know that?" I asked slowly while I remembered my struggle even to want to visit with him.

"My friend told me. Are you glad it's Christmas?"

"I am," I responded, momentarily wondering who his friend was. "I love Christmas."

"Me, too. Does that hurt? It looks like it hurts a lot. I'll bet it does, doesn't it?"

Glancing down, I saw that Fred was pointing at the blackened nail of my left forefinger, smashed when we were moving months before. I was startled that he had noticed it but even more startled at the genuine concern and even pain that filled his voice.

"No," I quickly told him, "it doesn't hurt. It did once, but no more."

"Oh, that's good," he breathed with relief. "I hate to hurt. I fell once and hurt my head. It was awful. My friend says I have limitations. Do you know what limitations are?"

Once again caught off-guard, I struggled to formulate an answer. "Uh . . . why don't you tell me," I finally suggested.

Fred nodded agreement. "Limitations are when I can't do all the things that other people do," he stated quickly. "I have limitations here in my head. But my friend told me that as long as I have a really warm spirit, my limitations won't matter. Then after I die I won't have limitations anymore. Does the bus go past your house?"

"Uh . . . the bus? No, I . . . uh . . ."

"I have an apartment of my own, and I ride the bus up here to work. When I hurt my head it was because I fell off the step of the bus. The snow made it slick. Does that hurt?"

Again I looked down to where he was pointing, and this time Fred had spotted a small scab on my other hand, a scab I had not even realized was there. Gently his forefinger was touching it.

"No," I replied as I shook my head in wonder. "I don't even remember hurting it."

"That's good," he said, definite relief once again sounding in his voice. "It isn't fun to hurt. My friend says that if I can keep my warm spirit, after I die I won't ever hurt again. If a warm spirit is caused by love, why isn't your spirit as warm as mine?"

I don't think I even answered him that time. The question was too direct, too abrupt, and the answer was too painful.

"Here," he said, I believe sensing my discomfort, "let me feel your spirit again. See? It's getting warmer—a little. My friend says that means that you are getting more love. Do you have someone in the hospital you are visiting?"

"Yes," I replied as I pulled my hand back to feel it for warmth that I truly hoped was there. "My baby daughter is upstairs. She . . . has limitations, too. In fact, when she was born, God didn't give her all she needed in order to live. Now she is slowly dying."

"Then she has a *really* warm spirit, doesn't she."

"Yes," I said quietly, "I suppose she does."

"Did you know that Jesus has the warmest spirit of all?"

"I . . . hadn't ever thought of it . . . like that."

"He does. My friend told me so."

More and more I was admiring the wise counsel of this unnamed friend, a person I would likely never know. But oh, the wonderful labor he was performing with this young man named Fred—and, through Fred, with others.

"You love your friend, don't you," I said.

"I love everybody," Fred replied simply.

I didn't know how to respond to such a sweeping declaration of righteousness, especially when it was made with such sincerity. So I did the only thing I could do—I changed the subject.

"What do you like best about Christmas?"

Fred looked at me as though he were contemplating an answer, though I was soon to learn that such was not the case. Instead, he threw me another curve.

"Did you know that Jesus came to the hospital today?" he abruptly asked.

"Huh? I mean . . . Jesus *what?*"

Fred gazed at me soberly. "Jesus came to the hospital," he repeated matter-of-factly. "For his birthday. It's Christmas, you know. Christmas is for celebrating Jesus' birthday. My friend says I will have a family of my own after I die, that I can have Christmas with. That's because I won't have limitations anymore. Why do you think Jesus came to the hospital?"

"Uh . . . I . . . uh . . . Why . . . uh . . . would you think?" I asked, for the first time in the conversation seeing no recourse but to take the offensive.

"Oh," he said, still very serious, "I already told you, but I just wondered if you heard. He came because it's Christmas, and he wanted to help us celebrate his birthday. He came down here in the kitchen to see me, too."

"He did?" I asked, no longer surprised by anything this young man might say. "I . . . uh . . . how do you know that?"

Fred looked at me seriously. "He loves me, you know. He is my friend. That is why my spirit is so warm today. I think when he came to see me and wish me Merry Christmas and Happy Birthday, he gave me some of his warm spirit to help mine be warmer. If the bus ever comes to your house, can I come see you?"

"Why . . . uh . . . certainly," I replied, still trying to comprehend Fred's simple but practically incomprehensible claim. "I'd like that."

For a moment or so Fred ate in silence, but I ate nothing. I believe I toyed with my food a little, but my mind was racing too much to eat. This young man actually believed that Jesus had come to the hospital. *This* hospital! On *this day!* For some crazy reason he thought that Jesus had come to the—

Suddenly I sat straight up, feeling as if my mind might explode with one overwhelming question. The incredible inner warmth and sense of love and peace that my wife and I had felt during the church service—might that have been related to the event that Fred was telling me he had experienced?

"Fred," I questioned as I struggled to understand, to believe, "what . . . what time do you think . . . I mean, what time did Jesus come?"

"A little while ago," he answered after politely clearing his mouth of food. "This morning, just before everybody came to eat. This is good gravy."

I nodded agreement, but my mind was still scrambling, trying to believe, first, that Jesus' immortal presence might have actually come to this place; and second, that what my wife and I had experienced might have been at least a tiny portion of the same transcendent event. I would never have imagined such a thing—could not have! Not, at least, until Fred's quietly confident statement. Now, as I forced my mind to consider something that I am sad to say I would ordinarily have scoffed at, I suddenly realized that a passage of scripture from the New Testament was going through my mind, around and around as if it were on a drum. I was thinking: " . . . but Jesus hid himself . . . going through the midst of them, and so passed by" (John 8:59).

Occasionally during his mortal ministry, I remembered reading in some commentary or other, Jesus had passed completely unnoticed through crowds of people, both large and small. That ability or power had been especially important, the commentary had continued, when the throngs of individuals had been antagonistic or without faith, and it simply hadn't been time for them to take his life.

If he had been in the presence of others without being seen when he was mortal, I thought next, how much simpler it would be for him to accomplish the same thing today! *But wait just a cotton-picking minute!* my doubting mind screamed in a last, desperate assault of mortal logic, what was I *thinking?* Who was I, that I could even for one moment consider the possibility that Kathy and I might have been privy to such a supernal moment? Or who was this truly innocent but nevertheless "limited" young man, that he could so matter-of-factly pro-claim it? Finally, who were any of us to have the temerity to imagine that a God, resurrected and eternal, would actually come from the heavenly realms to spend a few moments of real time mingling in a real place with a number of real people? The very idea seemed ludicrous, maybe even blasphemous. It was . . .

It was what? my limited faith questioned, gently reasserting itself. Why was I questioning the power of God? Was there anything that Jesus could not do? Surely he really does love and care for us as much today as he did those few people in Palestine nearly 2,000 years ago. Surely he would desire to minister to the terrible needs of some of his sweet, pure, innocent ones who were suffering so much pain, little tattered angels such as my daughter. Surely he had manifested his love in one form or another to many people in the hospital that day.

Surely—

"I'm very careful on the steps of the bus," Fred declared, breaking into my thoughts as though we had never even spoken of anything else. "That's because I don't want to hurt my head anymore. I'll be careful when I come to see you. Are you through eating?"

Dumbly I nodded.

"I can't go upstairs where the babies are, but I can walk up and down the hall. Can I walk to the bottom of the stairs with you?"

I nodded again. We picked up our trays, and in silence we handed them through the window to another dishwasher. Then we turned and walked down the hall to the foot of the stairs.

"Would you let me shake your hand?" Fred asked as we paused.

Eagerly I took his hand, and was surprised at the firmness of his grip. The firmness and the warmth.

"Can I shake your other hand?"

Somewhat awkwardly I shook his other hand.

"Your spirit is getting warmer," he said, encouraging me along just as I used to encourage my children when they were small. "Can I have a hug?"

Silently I nodded, and so Fred put his arms around me and pulled me close. Then he held me, his cheek pressed tightly against mine. After what seemed to me a long time, he pulled away and looked at me.

"Your spirit is much warmer than it was. When you hug me, does it make you nervous?"

"Why?" I asked, feeling guilty because it had.

"Some people don't like to hug. They think it is bad. But they don't have very warm spirits. I like you a lot. Can I have another hug?"

We hugged again, shook hands twice more, and, still without a smile, Fred told me that he loved me. That was when I decided to ask him.

"Fred, do you ever wish you didn't have . . . limitations? I mean, do you ever think you got handed a raw deal in life? Don't you get tired of things being so hard all the time?"

His countenance very serious, Fred regarded me in silence. In fact, he was quiet so long that I wondered if he had even understood my questions. I was about to ask them again, using different words, when he finally responded.

"When I hurt my head, I told my friend that hurting was very hard. He told me that when things got hard for me, it just meant that Jesus loved me lots."

"But wouldn't Jesus want to help you—to stop your pain?"

"Hurting *does* help me," Fred answered with absolute certainty. "It helps me to feel like Jesus felt when he hurt. My friend said that all Jesus' life he had hard things happen to him, just like I do. He told me to remember that Jesus wasn't born in a nice hospital like this one, but in a barn. He was wrapped in ragged old clothes, and they made his bed out of a smelly place where animals ate."

Jesus, too, had been tattered, I realized with surprise. Jesus Christ had also been tattered—

"If Jesus hadn't hurt a whole bunch, more even than me, my friend says he couldn't have been my Savior." Fred paused, looking at me. "But even when he hurt, Jesus was always happy. My friend says I should be happy, too; happy I have been blessed to be like Him. That's why I'm happy. I'm always happy!"

"And your limitations?" I pressed. "Don't you wish you didn't have them?"

"If I didn't have limitations," Fred declared slowly, patiently, I believe making sure that I understood, "I wouldn't have such a warm spirit. That would make it much harder for me to be Jesus' friend. I'm happy I'm his friend, because today he came to see me and wish me Merry Christmas and Happy Birthday."

Then, without another word, Fred turned and walked away.

Silently I stood watching him, trying my best to sort out the incredible array of emotions I was experiencing, the deep understanding I felt I was being given. Fred was happy in his limitations—in being a tattered angel—because that helped him be more like Christ Jesus. He did not think he had been given a raw deal!

And suddenly I knew, if I could have spoken with tiny Charity—if I could have just talked with her for five minutes about her seemingly unfair pain and suffering—she would have told me the same thing. "It is worth it!" she would have said with one of her sweetest smiles. "It is worth every agonizing moment I will ever be called upon to endure."

Filled with rejoicing that perhaps I now understood a little of God's love for his tattered angels, and perhaps something as well of his reason for allowing them to suffer, I was just turning to hurry up the stairs when the voice of my new friend spun me back around. "Someday when the bus comes to your house," Fred called out from halfway down the hall, "I will come to see you. Then I can feel your little girl's warm spirit, and she can feel my warm spirit. She has limitations like mine, so Jesus loves her a lot, just like he loves me. My friend says that limitations are what make us special to him. I'll bet Jesus came to wish your little girl Happy Birthday too."

As Fred spoke so matter-of-factly of what he surely believed was Christ's visit, I thought once again of my feelings from earlier in the day, my overwhelming sense of warmth and love. And suddenly I understood the most important thing of all about God's tattered angels, his imperfect and suffering sons and daughters.

"Yes," I replied softly, "I'm sure he loves Charity too, and it wouldn't surprise me to learn someday that he did visit her today. In fact, I'm sure that somehow he wished a Merry Christmas and Happy Birthday to everybody—every single one of his tattered angels.

"Thank you, Fred, for helping this one to see."

And then, filled at long last with the beginnings of the hope in Christ that surpasses understanding and makes *all* things bearable, I turned and flew two steps at a time toward my precious wife and daughter.

Until I'm Ready

"Honey, what do you think she meant?"

It was nearly midnight, February 19, 1990, the end of a long day that seemed also like the end of a long year and a half. Not only had we been dealing almost constantly with sweet little Charity's problems, but our eldest daughter, Tami, had met a man, fallen in love, become engaged, and then abruptly called off her wedding five days before it was to have taken place.

Though such things are not supposed to happen to young women in love, Tami had discovered that her trust had been tragically misplaced. Kathy and I were enormously relieved that her discovery had come before the wedding instead of afterward, but of course Tami was personally devastated, and so the rest of us were awash in her pain.

It had been nearly two months since our overwhelming spiritual experience at Primary Children's Medical Center. I don't know what I had expected would happen after that—maybe a miraculous healing for Charity. Certainly I had secretly hoped for such a thing. Instead, Charity had grown rapidly worse once we had taken her home again after Christmas, and in January we had been forced to hospitalize her for ten more days with another shunt replacement, her tenth, and antibiotics to combat a dangerous infection.

In other words, life with Charity continued as unpredictably as ever.

101

No matter how hard I prayed, no matter what I thought the Lord would surely do next in behalf of our tattered little angel, I was always surprised. More and more I found myself contemplating the words of the prophet Isaiah: "For my thoughts are not your thoughts, neither are your ways my ways, saith the Lord. For as the heavens are higher than the earth, so are my ways higher than your ways, and my thoughts than your thoughts" (Isaiah 55:8–9). Certainly I had learned that God's thoughts and ways were beyond my comprehension—especially, it seemed, as they pertained to our adopted daughter.

Staring up through the darkness toward the ceiling, I shook my head, trying to focus my thoughts. "I don't know what she meant, Kath. Say it again, just as you remember it."

Sighing with concern, Kathy leaned back into her pillow. *"Please don't be worried about me, Mom,"* she repeated quietly. *"I'm not going to die until I'm ready."*

"You're sure it was Charity who was speaking?"

"Yes, I'm sure."

"Did you hear her voice with your ears, or in your mind?"

"Blaine, why does it matter?" Kathy was beginning to sound frustrated with me. "Anyway, I'm certain it was in my mind. But the important thing is, what did she mean? That's what I don't understand."

As the light from Charity's bedroom filtered down the hall and into ours, I pondered my wife's question. Charity could not tolerate darkness even in her sleep, and was continually restless unless a light was left on in her room. Yet still, I marveled, there were those who insisted that she could not see, could not hear, could not feel, could not possibly respond to any stimuli in any way.

"I don't know what she could have meant," I finally answered. "She's finally feeling good, and seems to be past all of her crises. If she thought we were worried about her possibly dying, you'd think she would have given us this message months ago when her flurry of failed shunts and surgeries began."

"Unless," Kathy breathed, "there's something else coming—something worse than anything we've yet faced."

"I hope you're wrong!"

"Me too." In the silence that followed, our bedside monitor picked up the quiet whispering of the Kangaroo pump in Charity's room as it slowly fed liquids into our sleeping daughter—that and the ticking of the clock on her bedroom wall. Yet she was sleeping so peacefully that we could not even hear her breathing. It was the best she had slept—the best she had felt—in months. So why would she give us such a dire warning?

We found out why just three weeks later, as we sat across the desk from the doctor. His tenderly spoken words, "Your daughter is dying," had quite literally taken our breath away. "She cannot live longer than another . . . oh, four days, at the very most," he continued, doing his best to help us understand.

"What . . . do you think we should do?" It was Kathy speaking, and I could tell that this had hit her with terrible force.

"My recommendation," the doctor responded kindly, "is that we pull the shunt, stop her antibiotics, and discontinue everything but her seizure medications and food. Then we should release her from the hospital so you can take her home to be with her family. I think all of you would feel more comfortable having her there, and I'm certain she would feel the same."

"Are you positive she's dying?" I pressed.

"Yes, I am." Pausing, the doctor gazed down at our little girl, his countenance betraying both his emotion and his affection. "You know," he finally declared as he caressed her tiny hand and arm, "I've really grown to love this little girl. I am so amazed that she has overcome the odds and lived this long. I never thought she would do it. The fact that she has is a miracle I attribute totally to the love you two have given her." Again he paused, thinking. "I just wish I knew of something else we could do, some super antibiotic we could administer that would destroy this infection. But I don't, and there is nothing stronger than what we have tried."

Turning, he looked back at us. "Despite our best efforts, Charity has not responded to antibiotics, she is vomiting and has diarrhea continually, and her spinal fluid has become so thickened with the meningitis infection that even her exterior shunt is completely blocked. You can see for yourselves that the fluid has turned to jelly. This morning I directed one of the nurses to attempt to withdraw fluid directly from inside her skull in order to ease the pressure, and it had become too thick even for that.

"Your daughter isn't responding to anything we have done, and her condition continues to deteriorate. The four days I have given her, of course, are only a guess. Her death might occur a day or so sooner or later, but it will occur nonetheless. It is only a matter of time."

While my mind whirled with unanswered and probably unanswerable questions, Kathy pressed forward. "So you're asking for what, then? Our permission?"

"That's right, Kathy. I'd like your permission to discontinue all medical procedures except the ones I mentioned, and to release little Charity from PCMC to the care of your family."

"Do you need an answer right now?"

"Of course not." The doctor smiled sympathetically. "I know this is a terrible decision to face, and I don't blame either one of you for wanting to think it through. Why don't you take some time this after-noon? Go off alone somewhere and talk it over, and then let me know what you decide. And remember, if you feel that we should keep try-ing no matter how bleak her condition seems, that is exactly what we will do."

A little later Kathy and I were in the car, driving aimlessly south-ward until we somehow found ourselves in an area we had discovered years before—a secluded place of quiet beauty where we could talk and pray together.

"I just don't understand it!" I declared angrily. "Why would Charity go to all the trouble of warning us not to worry if she was just going to pass away three or four weeks later?"

"I . . . I don't know." Kathy was having a difficult time speaking. "I feel so torn, Blaine. I can't bear to see her suffering, and yet I can't stand the thought of her passing away—oh, what would I ever do without her?"

For a time we sat in silence, each of us absorbed in our own thoughts, our own memories. I thought of Kathy's remarkable experi-ence, of the fever that had seemed to strike Charity out of nowhere the next day—a fever so pronounced that Kathy had called Mary Bushman, our home health-care nurse. Upon checking Charity's heart rate and temperature, Mary had insisted that we leave immediately for the emer-gency room at Primary Children's Medical Center—a recommendation she had never before made.

At PCMC a series of tests had been run, and in a short time we had been informed that Charity had contracted spinal meningitis and that they were admitting her immediately. The nearly three weeks since then seemed nothing but a blur of medical procedures, beginning with a shunt replacement, Charity's eleventh. But because the tenth shunt had been contaminated by the meningitis (and had possibly been the contaminating agent that had given her the infection in the first place), Charity's new shunt had been placed externally, left on the outside of her little body so hospital personnel could more readily monitor Charity's spinal fluid.

She had also been placed on continuous doses of antibiotics, which were increased in strength or changed altogether as the days passed and it became obvious they were not doing their job. And finally she had been connected by wires and tubes to various monitors and other devices, none of which seemed to be doing anything but providing further bad news.

With the daily visits of one or more of our adult children, each painfully aware of their precious little sister's condition, and with our own day-to-day discouragements, the mood in our home had become terribly somber. We prayed for Charity, of course, but it was growing increasingly difficult to know what to pray for. Was it selfish of us to want her to live? Were we trying through our faith to thwart God's will? We didn't know, but these were issues we had been dealing with even before the doctor's painful announcement and recommendation.

"Kath," I finally asked as we sat together that March afternoon, "what do *you* think we should do?"

Instantly Kathy burst into a new flood of tears, and as I tried to comfort her I did the same.

"This is so hard," she finally said when a little control had returned. "Why can't Heavenly Father make the decision for us? Why do *we* have to be the ones who decide?"

"I . . . don't know. I just know that by tonight we have to go back and give the doctor some sort of direction."

"Do you have any feelings?"

"Millions of them," I sighed, "and all of them are painful. I'm just like you, Kath. I can't even begin to imagine our home without little Charity in it! Who would have thought that a severely handicapped little kid who can't do anything but smile would find a way to work herself into our hearts the way Charity has?"

For several minutes both of us were silent, thinking of the practically endless ways we felt love and joy whenever we were in Charity's presence, and wondering that it had so soon come to an end. Finally, then, we prayed together.

"I believe," Kathy whispered a little later as she wiped more tears from her eyes, "that despite our desire to keep her with us, we should do as the doctor suggests. I don't want to be the cause of Charity suffering any longer than she has to."

"I agree," I said, though a question nagged at the back of my mind.

An hour or so later, back in the hospital, we gave the doctor our decision.

"I'm certain that's the best thing you can do for her," he responded quietly.

"We think so too," I agreed. "But now I have a question. What happens if she doesn't die?"

"She will die, Blaine. She is dying right now."

I nodded. "I know that. But what happens if the process is somehow stopped, and she lives for, say, a few more months or even years?"

"It won't happen."

"But suppose it does," I persisted, reluctant to share my overwhelming feeling—one that had come during our prayer together earlier—that Charity's message to Kathy had been for now, and that she was not yet going to die. "Suppose she gets better on her own. Will we put in another shunt, or what?"

The doctor shook his head. "This little girl has suffered enough. I would not want to consider putting her through more of these surgeries, and I would hope you wouldn't. So, no. No more shunts.

"Now, it's too late to get Charity ready tonight, so why don't you folks both go home and get a good rest. When you come back in the morning we'll have her ready for you. I'm certain she will enjoy spending her last few days with her family."

"You're probably right," I acknowledged. "Except that I don't think she's ready to die just yet—"

CHARITY'S PARTY

◆

That night, after the shunt, IVs and every other external device except the Kangaroo pump had been removed from Charity's body, the strangest thing happened. One of the nurses, coming in to check on Charity, dropped her stethoscope on the floor. When she exclaimed something or other in exasperation, Charity began to giggle. Astonished that this deathly ill little child without a brain could respond in such a normal and joyful way, the nurse hurried out and told others. They came to see for themselves, were just as amazed by Charity's continued smiles and giggles, and left to further spread the word. By the time we arrived the next morning to take her home, several people were anxious to tell us of the party Charity had held in her room—a party that had ended only an hour or so before our arrival.

Some of these people, including one or two of the doctors who had dropped in to observe for themselves, had refused until that night to believe our descriptions of Charity's incredible ability to respond to us. Yet after those few hours of Charity's joyful party they had to believe, for they had seen for themselves what they thought had been nothing more than the wishful thinking of two doting parents who were trying to make their brainless daughter come to life.

Charity *could* laugh, she could tell when people were near, she could respond to them, she could—well, suffice it to say that we found ourselves in the amazing position of listening as *others* tried to convince *us* of our daughter's unbelievable abilities.

Though there was never an official attempt made by the medical profession to explain Charity's remarkable behavior that night, one of the doctors suggested, and both Kathy and I felt he was right, that it was nothing more nor less than a night of rejoicing for our little angel. We believe she knew that her eleventh shunt would be her last, that her surgeries and even her stays in the hospital—which now totaled ninety-three days out of her eighteen short months of life—would also be her last. She was through with those things forever! She had run that particular race, passed the test, and endured to the end. Whatever time she had left in mortality, she would spend it surrounded by her own family, her loved ones. To us it was no wonder that she spent a few hours rejoicing and sharing her happiness and gratitude with those who had tried so diligently to make her life a little more bearable.

March was about two-thirds gone when we took Charity home to be with our family, and both Kathy and I took immediate steps to arrange a funeral and notify friends and loved ones that Charity was dying. Any good-byes, we told everyone, needed to be accomplished within the next two or three days. Many who had learned to love our little angel came, and they left in tears, convinced they would not see her again until the hereafter.

Despite her night of happiness, Charity continued to struggle, trembling with pain, crying frequently, breathing with ragged gasps, and suffering continual bouts of nausea and tissue-destroying diarrhea. For Kathy and me those were a couple of long days and nights as we spent every possible moment with our suffering little angel. My feeling that she was not about to die wouldn't leave, but I couldn't believe it any longer. Charity had grown incredibly pale and weak, and there were simply too many things wrong with her for me to imagine that she could survive.

On the afternoon of her third day at home, with our parents, our children, and a few others crowded into Charity's bedroom, I carefully laid my hands upon her shorn and battered little head and tearfully bid her farewell. In my prayer I told her that although each of us loved her and hated to see her go, we were all thrilled that she would finally be released from her suffering little body and could return to be with Jesus.

I ended my prayer and then stepped back to hold my grieving wife as we waited for our daughter's death. But nothing happened. There seemed to be a brief pause in Charity's breathing, a few seconds, perhaps, and then all continued as before. After an hour or so, we realized that she hadn't cried since the blessing. By the next morning there was a noticeable change in her breathing: it wasn't so labored, so ragged. She had stopped vomiting, we realized the following afternoon, and in another day or two, when her diarrhea also stopped, we began to feel hope.

A Sweet Healing

"Dad, are you awake?"

Tami's voice, despite the fact that it was barely loud enough to hear, sounded urgent. Easing myself out of bed, I fumbled with my glasses and then glanced at the clock. Just after 4:00 A.M. For an instant I listened to Kathy's deep and regular breathing, feeling thankful that she was asleep. In the past year and a half there had hardly been a night when she had slept all night long—

"Dad! Wake up, please!"

Quietly I put on my robe and moved through our door and into Charity's room, where I knew Tami would be waiting.

"I didn't want to wake Mom. That's why I was trying to hold my voice down."

"She's still asleep, Sis, so you did fine. What's wrong?"

Instantly Tami's tired-looking eyes filled with tears, and both of us looked to the little child cradled in her arms. "Charity's worse again, Dad. She's arching her neck terribly, her whole body's trembling, and I can't keep the phlegm suctioned out of her throat."

"You sure?"

Wiping her eyes, Tami nodded. "I am. I think she's even worse than a month ago, when the doctor said the meningitis was still there and that she was still dying. Dad, does this make sense to you? That Charity would take two months to die?"

It was a fair question, and one I had no idea how to answer. It had now been sixty days since we had discontinued all antibiotics and other heroic measures to keep Charity alive, and had brought her home from PCMC to die in peace. Despite this well-intentioned abandonment, however, Charity had continued clinging to life with a tenacity that befuddled everyone, us included.

Though she had neither smiled nor laughed in those two months, most of the time Charity had seemed at least somewhat peaceful. But four weeks earlier she had begun stressing, clenching her little fists, pressing her arms against her chest, trembling throughout her body, and struggling for breath. That had continued for a few days and stopped. Now she was doing it again.

Fortunately, after Charity's hospital stay at Christmas, the doctors had prescribed a sedative. It helped Charity a great deal, and except during her worst times we could usually count on her getting three to four hours of uninterrupted sleep. But we had also learned that even the sedative didn't much affect her when her body was struggling, as it now was. And sedated or not, Charity had to have the phlegm suctioned from her throat, the Kangaroo pump monitored, and so forth. She had become a twenty-four-hour-care baby.

"Dad," Tami suddenly said as she held up her Bible, which she had been reading almost constantly of late, "listen to this." She then read St. Paul's definition of charity from the New Testament—the same verses I had felt guided to when selecting Charity's name nearly two years before.

"I cannot imagine a better description of Charity," Tami continued as she lowered the book. "This little angel is the perfect embodiment of Paul's words. You know, Dad, I believe Charity absolutely loves the Lord Jesus Christ, and I believe she is beloved of him. She radiates his love, and I'm really starting to feel it."

"I know you are, Tam," I replied. "And I'm sure she's feeling your love, too. Now, why don't you let me take Charity, and you get some rest. Then when Mom wakes up we'll take the poor little angel back to the emergency room at PCMC and see if they can determine what else we might do."

"Nothing has changed," Kathy said with discouragement a few hours later as we drove home from PCMC. "After two months the spinal meningitis is still there, and they are still convinced that Charity's brain stem has been damaged beyond recovery and she is dying." She began to weep again. "Blaine, I'm scared! They really don't want anything more to do with us. They as much as told us that today."

"Actually," I tried to explain, "what they said was that they still didn't feel we should consider any more shunts or other heroic measures, Kath. And we agreed to that two months ago."

"I know we did. But . . . but what if she lives for a year or more, and her head pressures return? I couldn't stand that! I couldn't stand seeing her suffer again!"

"She isn't even crying anymore, Kath. In fact, do you realize she hasn't made a sound of any sort in two months?"

"I . . . know." Kathy removed her hand from under Charity's legs where she was holding her, and wiped at her eyes. "Mostly, I think that's because she's comatose."

"Well, maybe today she is," I argued. "But you know how responsive she's been to Tami these past few weeks. Especially her eyes. Tami says she can watch Charity's eyes and practically tell what she is trying to say. That doesn't happen when she's comatose."

"You're right," Kathy replied with a sigh. "It doesn't. But she's definitely comatose right now."

"Then I don't think it will last long," I stated confidently.

"Why not?"

I smiled. "Because I think Charity has decided, somehow, to stay alive long enough to help her big sister recover from her broken heart. Or rather, the Lord has allowed her to stay. If I'm right, it doesn't make sense that she would spend her time being unconscious."

For a moment Kathy gazed out the window of the car. "I didn't know if you'd noticed," she finally breathed. "How much Charity is affecting Tami, I mean."

"A person would have to be blind not to notice. Not that I blame her, you understand, but Tami was terribly withdrawn after her wedding plans blew up in her face."

"It didn't help that we'd been trying for months to warn her that something didn't feel right about it," Kathy said tenderly.

"I know. No young adult alive wants to be wrong in such an important decision, especially in front of her parents. Anyway, I'm amazed at how rapidly Tami is softening, becoming her tender, loving self again. Because she hasn't found a job, she's spending all these hours with Charity, helping both her and you in a way we never thought anyone could. And while she's doing that, Charity's love is quickly softening and refilling her heart."

And so it was. Tami's closeness to her sweet baby sister continued to grow stronger, and she sought every opportunity to be with her. Like others who had felt Charity's love, including us, Tami seemed never able to get enough of it, and it definitely had an impact on her.

This is how Tami described those days: "I'm frightened sometimes when I wonder what my life would have been like without Charity.

After my ex-fiancé flew home in February 1990 I felt displaced, alone, and very unsure of my identity as well as my self-worth. They say that man's extremity is God's opportunity, and that was certainly true for me. The Lord, in his infinite wisdom, loved me enough to provide a way for my soul to be healed. For three months I was unable to find work, and during that time he gave me the gift of my sweet angel sister, Charity.

"Day after day I would rock her, sing to her, bare my soul to her, and frequently cry as I held her close. I've often said that holding her was like holding love, for she demanded nothing but gave everything. Day after day my wounds grew less and less painful until my heart began to feel again. And then I found a job. On my second day at work, May 2, 1990, I met a young man named David Bestenlehner, who almost immediately asked me to go out with him. On our first date I took David home and introduced him to my sweet little sister. He loved her from the instant he met her, and it was easy to see that she loved him. As I watched them together I had some very strong feelings, and I *knew* that the hand of the Lord was indeed directing my life."*

Our family never stopped feeling overwhelmed by Charity's ability to give pure love–without asking or even hoping for anything in return. It was not only a miracle that she was still alive, but it seemed an even greater miracle that she was still able to reach out and tenderly soothe us with her love. Perhaps, we were beginning to conclude, this was the very reason why God had spared her life.

---

* David and Tami were married exactly one year later, on May 2, 1991.

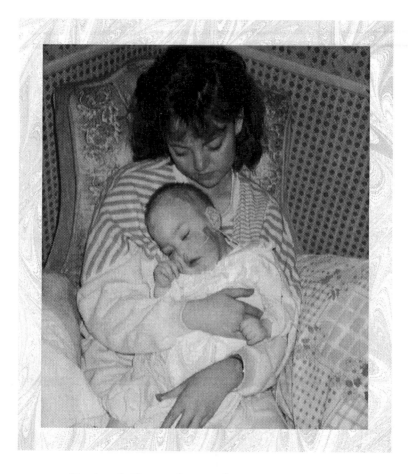

Tami and Charity during Charity's seven-month
ordeal with spinal meningitis.

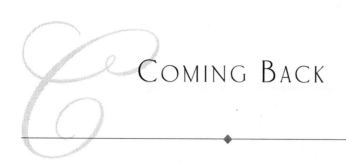

COMING BACK

"Blaine! Blaine, come quick!"

I ran for Charity's room, prepared for goodness only knew what the next catastrophe might be. "What is it? What's wrong?"

Kathy held her finger to her smiling lips. "Sshhh. Don't frighten or startle her. Just listen."

It was now the first part of September, 1990, and Charity had not only just passed her second birthday but had lived seven months beyond her spinal meningitis—seven months longer than anyone had expected she could. She was now lying quietly on top of the two mattresses in her crib (built up to ease the strain on Kathy's back), her dancing eyes darting rapidly back and forth.

"What am I listening for?" I whispered.

"You'll see," Kathy said, stepping back from the crib. "Lean down and quietly tell her good morning."

Wondering, I leaned close to Charity's little face. "Good morning, punkin-doodle," I murmured, using my personal favorite of Charity's nicknames. Tami had come up with the name Chare-bear, which most of the family had adopted. But me, I still liked punkin-doodle, punkin-doo, and squirt.

"Good morning, Charity," I repeated, resisting the urge to lean closer and begin smothering her with kisses. "Are you hiding somewhere in that cute little body? If you are, come out, come out, wherever you are."

For an instant Charity's eyes grew wide with surprise and recognition. Then, to my delight and astonishment, her face opened into one of the most beautiful smiles I have ever seen. It was also the first one I had seen from her in seven long months.

"Well, good morning," I beamed as I kissed her on the bridge of her nose. "Thank you for that beautiful smile, punkin-doo. Seeing it makes Mommy and me so happy!"

I straightened up to wipe the sudden tears from my eyes, tears of happiness and gratitude that I didn't want splashing onto her. However, a tear escaped my hand and hit her face, and that was when Charity started to giggle. Apparently she had been giggling earlier with Kathy, but now as I watched her little body shake with her vigorous, deep-voiced chuckling, I knew with certainty that she was back. Whatever had happened, whatever damage had been done by the meningitis, it had been mended through the power of God and the marvelous self-healing abilities of the human body.

It had been a long seven months, but now our little angel was back with us, smiling and laughing with Kathy and me just like on her good days from before.

Off and on for about an hour Charity laughed and played, and I don't know that I have ever felt greater joy. I laughed with her, I tickled and nuzzled her, Kathy and I sang a dozen or more songs to her, and we both wept almost constantly as we watched our tattered little angel, who had literally been snatched from the dead, respond to our antics so delightfully.

As she finally settled down and went to sleep, I reflected on her smile, thinking of how overwhelmed I was by the incredible feeling of warmth and love that swept over me each time I saw it. And I knew again, as I had known from the first week or so that Charity had been in our home, that her smile was her way of saying, "Thank you!" and "I love you!"

Up and Down Cycles

◆

In spite of this remarkable improvement, life with Charity continued to be joy mixed with difficulty. From the latter part of 1990, when she came out of her seven-month ordeal, until the spring of 1993, she went through a lengthy series of ups and downs in her health that were baffling to everyone. Though not exactly predictable in their timing, these cycles could always be counted on to occur.

Kathy says: "I could tell Charity's health was in a deteriorating cycle, or as we put it, 'going downhill,' when she became tense instead of relaxed. She had a harder time smiling at me because she was obviously hurting or feeling discomfort. After a very short time—a few hours to a day or so—she would begin trembling along with being tense, and whimpering off and on. Her face would then take on the expression of a person who was in sheer agony, and she would try to move her head back, arching her back and neck. Sometimes it seemed almost impossible to get her body to straighten up, she would arch so badly. And she was very strong while she was arching, so much so that it was extremely difficult to hold her because of the pressure she applied to our arms.

"Under normal conditions, the pupils of Charity's eyes were so large that they appeared black rather than their natural, beautiful blue. As these periods of stress came on her, however, Charity's pupils would constrict down until they were little more than dark points, enabling us to see her bright, blue eyes. Unfortunately they also looked all glassed over, as if she weren't really in there. There would also be some bulging around her eyes, and her head would push back and back until her spine and neck were a complete arch.

"The final symptom or expression of Charity's down times was shallow, labored breathing, almost as though she were gasping for air. This was frightening for us to listen to, and was compounded by the perpetual mucous problem in her throat that required regular suctioning with a pump.

"This stressing and trembling and arching and labored breathing would go on for days and days, getting continually worse and leaving Charity unable to sleep at all because she was in so much discomfort. Even administering a sedative would only give her an hour or maybe two of sleep and peace, and then she would be awake and miserable again.

"Finally she would go comatose and seem to be gone from us entirely. During this time she would sleep deeply most of the time, day and night, except for brief moments when I changed her or cleaned her up. Then her eyes would flicker open and the look of pain would return. Though concerned, I was always relieved when she was comatose, for I knew that for however long it lasted, she was at least somewhat at peace.

"After three or four days of being comatose, she would wake up and go right back to where she had been before—agitated, trembling, suffering, and completely unable to sleep. This phase could go on for anywhere from three or four days to a week or more, and then she would gradually come out of this stress cycle and return to her relaxed, normal, and happy self. The whole downhill process usually lasted from seven to fifteen days, depending on the severity of the cycle.

"During Charity's bad days I slept very little, for I was constantly trying to make her more comfortable, experimenting with pillows, blankets, tilted mattresses, and anything else I could think of to try to help her little body relax. This was extremely frustrating, because what seemed to work one time would have the opposite effect the next. It was as if Charity was not about to follow any of the rules we thought she should follow.

"Of course that wasn't new, either. Though she wasn't supposed to grow, her growth was always near normal for her age. Though she wasn't supposed to hear, see, or process information, it was obvious that she could. Because she lacked a normal immune system, we continually expected her to come down with colds, flu, and the common childhood illnesses she was exposed to, yet besides the meningitis she never caught anything in her entire life but two or three small colds. She wasn't supposed to be able to recover on her own from spinal meningitis, but she did. Finally, she was never expected to feel anything physically, mentally, or emotionally. That was her biggest trick of all, for I am certain that she felt everything she ever encountered or experienced, probably more deeply than all the rest of us put together. No one who saw her smiles could remain unaffected by her joy; no one who saw her down times could doubt her suffering.

"Anyway, it made me so sad to see her feeling miserable, and often I would plead with the Lord to let me take the pain from her so she could have a little peace. Unfortunately, that never happened.

"When she came out of this downward cycle, she would have seven to fourteen or fifteen 'good days,' which we cherished dearly. During her good days she was completely relaxed and at peace. These were the times with Charity that I loved and enjoyed the most! I could always tell when she was coming out of her down spells because she would start giving me little smiles again in the midst of her suffering. These would grow more and more frequent and more and more dazzling as the hours and days went by, until she was once again fully responsive to everything that was going on around her. She would sing with me, talk to me in her own way, play what I called the 'Oooo' game as I made sounds that she did her best to imitate, track my movements about her bed with her dancing eyes, and completely wrap me around her soul and heart with her brilliant smiles. I'm not exaggerating when I say that each of her smiles brought tears to my eyes, and that I have never in my life felt greater joy and peace than while we were together during these up times."

Naturally Kathy and I were concerned when these cycles began, for they caused us to worry constantly. So far as we could tell, in each downward cycle Charity's spinal fluid was again increasing–the hydrocephalus or the "water on the brain" diagnosis she had carried since birth–increasing the pressure inside her little head and compressing her brain stem. Such a condition, we had learned early in her life as she staggered from one shunt surgery to the next, explained her bulging and constricted eyes, her arching neck and back, her labored breathing and comatose states, as well as her trembling and whimpering and all the classic evidences of the pain she was not supposed to feel.

The trouble was, each of these cycles was also supposed to be deadly, to be her very last. As we understood it, the hydrocephalic's body is not capable of relieving itself of excess spinal fluid, which is what moves upward and fills the skull of children like Charity. Hence the need for surgically implanted shunts to keep the head from swelling and the brain and/or brain stem from being damaged.

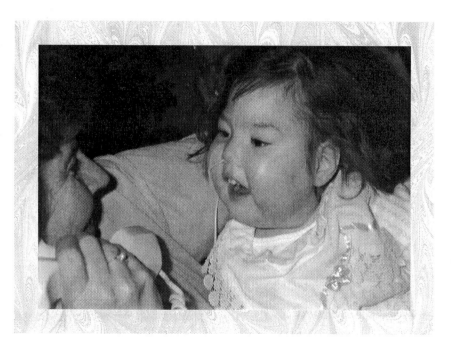

Kathy and Charity. On her "good days," Charity loved
to talk to her sisters on the telephone.

Because Charity no longer had a shunt, the theory was that her spinal fluid would steadily increase in volume until the pressure inside her head was sufficient to crush or destroy the brain stem, immediately killing her. And while it was happening we would see the symptoms Kathy has described above. As far as we know, this is why Charity's doctors were inclined again and again to predict her immediately impending death.

However, once more our daughter was apparently refusing to play by the medical rules. If she *was* experiencing increased spinal fluid and therefore head pressure during her down cycles, in her seven months of silence she had also found an internal and highly effective way of draining it back down. Thus she endured these almost monthly cycles, which continued without letup, until she was four and a half years old.

To Discomfort an Angel

$\diamond$

In the spring of 1991, during one of her "good times," Charity suddenly grew very ill. We couldn't tell what was wrong, the doctors couldn't tell, and even Tylenol and sedatives didn't bring her any peace. She was utterly miserable.

Of course, we prayed constantly for help in knowing what to do, but for a week we remained at a loss. Then one Saturday morning while I was pleading for her relief, it suddenly dawned on me that the problem might not be Charity's. Quickly I gathered the family in an emergency meeting.

"All right, listen up. You all know that Charity is doing badly. Since we can't seem to find a problem with her, I'm thinking that maybe the problem is with one of us."

"What are you talking about, Dad?"

"I'm talking about the fact that she is perfectly pure, without sin. Do you all agree with me?"

Everyone nodded.

"Okay, do you also agree that she will never, no matter how long she lives, have the capacity or desire to commit sin?"

"We all know that, Dad." Dan's mind was racing ahead, like always. "What's the point?"

I smiled. "The point is that Charity is truly a person of absolute purity, the only one I've ever known. And since sin and purity can't exist together, what do you suppose might happen if Charity was forced to be around sin?"

"She wouldn't like it," Michelle declared.

"How would she let us know she didn't like it? How would she react? Think about this, kids. Suppose one or more of us is doing something wrong. I don't mean the normal little stuff; I mean something pretty major that our conscience is already telling us we shouldn't be doing. With Charity being unable to get away from us because of her circumstances, and being unable to tolerate our sins because of her perfect purity, might her reaction be to get sick?"

Everybody looked at me in amazement, Kathy included.

"Remember," I went on, "I'm not suggesting that we need to be perfect. But I believe we each need to go off alone for a few minutes and search our souls. If I'm right, one of us is having a major problem with sin that we're hiding—but apparently we can't hide it from Charity, and it's hurting her. If it happens to be you, come tell me quickly, and let's get this taken care of before she suffers any further."

A few moments later one of the kids came quietly into my office, acknowledged a *very* inappropriate book hidden in the home, and asked what should be done. My instructions—and I was playing this completely by ear—were to take the book back to where it had come from, apologize to Charity, and then go off alone and apologize to God and seek his forgiveness.

My counsel was strictly followed, and thirty minutes later Charity was smiling and happy again, with no signs of her former illness about her.

Time and again in the months and years that followed, we observed this unnerving phenomenon. Charity reacted almost instantly to wickedness around her—she was not physically able to tolerate it. Though she loved being out with the family, if there was a lot of noise and commotion going on, especially arguing or bickering, it upset her terribly. She loved peaceful, quiet music such as hymns, but she could not tolerate anything loud or raucous. This sensitivity increased as she grew older. Except for occasional news broadcasts, she hated television, and would actually burst into tears when violence or evil—such as profanity, taking God's name in vain, and the crudeness and vulgarity of most current sitcoms and movies—was being portrayed.

On the other hand, she loved to have people stop by and visit her. These were happy times for Charity as she reached out and responded to them, loving them in a beautiful way. It was as though she exuded an aura of "goodness" that affected all who came near.

Barbara Evans, physical therapist for the school district where we lived for a time, recognized this trait of Charity's. She remembers: "After I had seen Charity several times, she began to recognize my voice and touch when I would start to talk to her or move her limbs, and she would respond to me. I soon couldn't wait for each week to pass so I could see her again. She was always so patient with me, and I felt so special that she knew my voice and touch, especially because when someone she did not know entered the room I could actually feel her body tension change. Then when they left she would relax again and allow me to continue range-of-motion therapy on her.

"When Charity was feeling good she could smile with her whole body (this sounds unreal but she could do this great trick) and make simple cooing sounds, and I would go away feeling so good, as if she had spoken a great thought to me. When I would visit and she didn't feel good I would feel down also, and would sorrow because she was having such a rough time. Even though Charity could not move her body or speak to me, she was able to communicate very clearly how she felt and that she knew me. She had a great spirit that I could actually feel."

The downside of this ability of Charity's occurred when individuals came into our home who were filled with unrighteousness. No matter what their problems might have been, almost immediately Charity began trembling, whimpering, and ultimately bursting into tears. Over time we grew brave enough to ask such visitors to leave, feeling that our daughter's well-being ought to be more important than their "ruffled feathers."

I wish I could say that it was mostly outsiders who brought such distress into Charity's life. Unfortunately that wasn't so, for we ourselves were usually the culprits. For instance, I have what some call a right-brained personality, often leaning more to emotion than good sense. Thus there were times when I became a great trial to little Charity.

One day I was speaking on the telephone with one of my close friends, whose personality is very similar to mine, and our conversation deteriorated into a disagreement. As my voice grew louder, I saw—and ignored–Kathy's vehement signals. I also ignored the fact that Charity was in her wheelchair only a few feet behind me, listening intently while her eyes widened with fear. For perhaps another thirty seconds I continued, my frustration obvious to all, and then, finally, I heard Charity's terrified whimpers. Turning, I watched in dismay as Kathy frantically disconnected her from her pump and rushed her back toward her bedroom. They had barely reached the hallway when Charity's whimpers became loud and anguished cries.

Sick at heart, I quickly apologized to my friend, excused myself, and offered up a mental apology to the Lord as I hurried to the side of my daughter. By then she was sobbing uncontrollably, but after maybe a

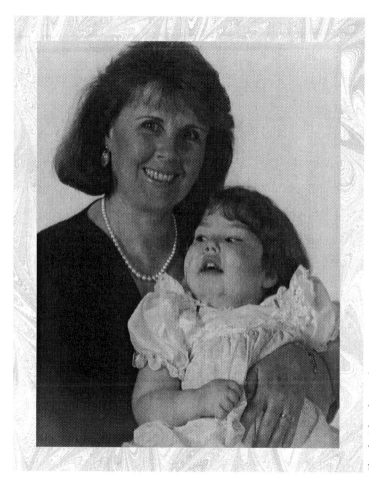

Kathy and Charity.

dozen of my tearful and heartfelt apologies to her and to her mother, she gradually regained control of herself. As I kissed her again and again she looked up at me, and with huge tears still in her beautiful eyes and on her cheeks, she smiled. *"I love you, Daddy,"* I knew she was saying with exquisite sweetness and infinite patience, *"but please try to do better. It hurts me when you don't."*

Charity also hated the way some of us in the family teased or put each other down, and she was quick to let us know how she felt. Gradually we managed to change those behaviors. She began crying if Kathy and I had a disagreement, especially if my voice grew loud. Even Dan and Michelle were able to see how their bickering caused her to feel pain.

Dan says: "When I think of Charity I also think of love. She hadn't been with our family very long before we realized the pain that our normal, everyday contentions caused her. Thus she helped us learn to love each other better, and in so doing we were showing the love we had for her. I can say without hesitation that Charity's coming into our lives is the single most important thing that has ever happened to our family."

Michelle adds: "Charity has touched and enriched my life in many ways. She emanates the sweetest spirit. Whenever I find myself struggling, in anything at all, I go to Charity's room because I know an angel resides there. Whatever my problem is, I can pick her up and hold her for a little while, and when I leave her room my problems always seem better. By reminding me to be a better person, she has taught me some of life's most important lessons, and I will always love her dearly."

Needless to say, having a little spiritual barometer in our home was a unique experience, occasionally highly discomforting, but always very beneficial.

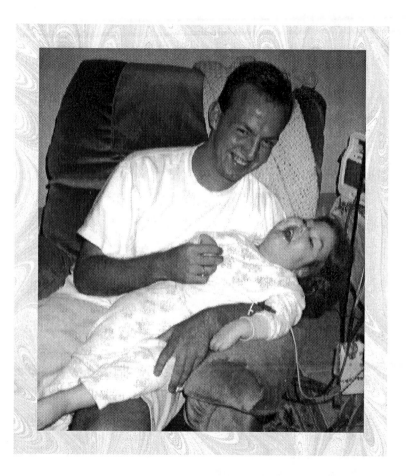

Charity enjoying a moment with her brother Dan.

CONTINUED COMMUNICATION

◆

"Dr. Tait's office returned your call," I said as I walked into Charity's room one morning in the summer of 1992, thinking of the wonderful neurologist who had always been such a friend to us and our daughter.

"Good." Kathy looked relieved. "Did you ask her about this new kind of seizure Charity has been having?"

Busy nuzzling Charity's cheek and neck and basking in her sweet joy, I did not immediately answer. "I tried," I finally said as I unclenched Charity's thumb and held her little hand, "but Dr. Tait wasn't on the line. However, the receptionist said they couldn't tell much until Dr. Tait could look at the medication levels in Charity's blood. They're making an appointment so we can take her into the hospital today and have some blood drawn."

Kathy gave me a long look of apprehension, and then moved around me so she could continue massaging the muscles in Charity's leg. One of the things most noticeable about our little girl was the amazingly translucent color of her skin. It was so clear and blemish-free—so porcelain-doll-like in its appearance—that it was almost startling to see. This was partly due to the fact that Charity did not get a lot of exposure to sunlight or the other elements, and partly because her blood vessels were tiny and were buried abnormally deep beneath the surface of her skin. This dramatically reduced the pink blush so evident in more normal children.

So far as we could tell, however, this presented no problems for Charity—except when it was time to draw blood. Then she suffered terribly as medical professionals probed again and again, sometimes a dozen or more times, searching with their needles for one of her well-hidden veins. We suffered with her as we watched, and I know the people attempting to draw the blood suffered as well. It is never pleasant watching a child in pain.

Charity endured such tests as well as she could, flinching and tensing more with each jab, and occasionally even whimpering. We would often go for months without ever hearing her cry, but eight or nine jabs with that needle were about all she could handle before the pain reduced her to tears. Sometimes the trauma was so great that it took her days to fully relax and become her happy self again.

That was why Kathy had looked so apprehensive.

An hour or so after the call from Dr. Tait's office, as we pulled out of the driveway to take Charity to the hospital, her smile, which we had been enjoying for days, abruptly vanished. Soon her body was tensing, and not long after that she started to whimper.

Concerned, I slowed and pulled to the side of the road so we could better see what might be hurting her. Finding nothing wrong, at least that we could see, and realizing that she had stopped whimpering, I started again toward the hospital.

Moments later the whimpering was back, and soon it escalated into full-fledged crying.

"What's wrong?" I asked as I glanced at Charity and then Kathy.

Shaking her head, Kathy looked as perplexed as I felt. "I don't know.

All her limbs are straight, the blanket isn't too tight, I know she isn't cold—I . . . well, I don't know what's wrong."

"Maybe she's trying to tell us something." I was thinking of how Charity reacted whenever we or the children had a serious argument.

"Maybe," Kathy replied as she tried to comfort our daughter, "but I don't know what it would be."

For another mile or so I continued driving, but by then Charity was sobbing so hard that both of us knew something awful must be happening. So once again I pulled the car to the side of the road.

"This is strange, Kath," I said after a second careful examination had proven futile. "She was fine when we left home, and now she's going to pieces. Nothing shows, but something is definitely wrong!"

"I . . . I know." Now Kathy was weeping along with our daughter. "But I don't know what it is!" Wiping her eyes with a corner of Charity's blanket, she looked at me. "Do you really think she's trying to tell us something?"

I nodded. "I don't think she wants this test, Kath. I'll bet anything she doesn't want to have her blood drawn."

Kathy sighed. "I think you're right."

"Then forget the test!" I said grimly. "Let's just turn around and take her home. If we're right, she'll stop crying as soon as we do."

"But what about her seizures? You said Dr. Tait's office has even called ahead to order the blood work they need."

"Who cares?" Carefully I turned the car and started back toward home. "Maybe Charity knows these new seizures aren't any big deal. Maybe she doesn't want more medication than she's already taking, no matter what the test results show. Maybe something's wrong we don't know about, and this trauma would push her over the edge. Maybe she simply doesn't want any more pain today. Maybe—"

"Honey, look."

Glancing over, I saw that Charity's cries were stopping, and that she was even trying to smile through her tears. Somehow I wasn't surprised. By the time we got back home she *was* smiling, with no more crying whatsoever, and both Kathy and I knew that this bright and articulate little girl who happened to have no physical brain had once again communicated most powerfully her desires and her needs.

A Major Change

"Charity, are you tricking Mommy again? Is that what you're doing, little munchkin? Are you getting sick again, or did you just get tired of sleeping and decide to have a party?"

It was early, before 5:00 A.M. on the last day of March, 1993, and both Kathy and I were up trying to figure out what to do with Charity. As far as we knew, she hadn't been asleep in nearly twenty-four hours, despite at least three doses of her sedative. At the moment she was smiling and appeared happy, but both of us knew that when she didn't sleep it usually meant she was starting into one of her down cycles. Usually. The trouble was, sometimes it didn't mean that. Whether it did or not, we seemed powerless to do anything about it anyway.

"Maybe she's just happy we're moving again," I ventured, thinking of the fact that our current rental home had just been sold and we needed to be renting somewhere else within a month. Kathy's look told me she thought I had lost it, and so I hastily explained that I hadn't meant to sound serious. No one liked to move, though since we had lost our home shortly after Charity's birth, moving from one rental to another had become a regular occurrence for us.

For the previous few weeks we had been house-hunting again—and had discovered to our dismay that due to a housing shortage there were no rentals available in our community or anywhere nearby.

Deciding to try to buy a small home, we had found one and put earnest money on it, only to have the owners call a day later with the news that someone had come along and given them an offer many thousands of dollars more than ours. They wanted us to either increase our offer or withdraw it so they could get what their home was really worth.

In the next two weeks that happened twice again, and so in desperation we hired a builder to construct a home for us in the Salt Lake Valley, where we would be much closer to Primary Children's Medical Center. The day we signed the contract, a home in the distant rural community of Fountain Green was made available to us to rent on a temporary basis. It would be Charity's fifth home since her birth, and four days later we were in it—a day ahead of our move-out date.

"Well," I said after our first night in our latest home, "it will be interesting to see why we've been moved here."

"I can't tell you why," Kathy said in frustration, "but I can tell you I just ran out of Charity's vitamins, and her prescription is in a pharmacy more than seventy miles away. This is not going to be fun, Blaine."

Circumstances did seem bleak, but we should have been bright enough to realize that nothing in Charity's life ever happened by accident. The Lord loved that little girl, and even if it had to be over our complaining bodies, he was about to perform a major miracle in her behalf.

Immediately we began to notice some changes. In the month since we had been told we needed to move, Charity's "bad days," or at least those caused by what we thought of as head pressures, had declined quite dramatically. Now those pressures stopped almost altogether, and day after day she seemed relaxed and peaceful. Just as amazing, despite the rural area in which we were living, Charity's terrible mucous problem appeared to be clearing up, and we went days at a time without having to suction the phlegm from her throat. This, we felt, was a direct answer to prayer, for we had pleaded with the Lord for years to help her breathe more freely.

It was almost three weeks before we were able to get a refill on Charity's vitamins, and to our surprise, when we began administering them she started filling up with mucous and her breathing problems returned. We immediately stopped the dosage, and within two or three days she was breathing freely again. Allergies! We would never have discovered this if we hadn't moved; thus our most difficult upheaval quickly became a blessing.

Fountain Green also provided Charity with some wonderful new friends. The day after our arrival we realized that two of the neighbor boys were jumping their four-wheelers over the elevated corner of our driveway, directly under Charity's window. They weren't hurting our driveway, but the noise of their machines terrified Charity and quickly reduced her to tears. After this had occurred several times, I went out and introduced myself to them, learning that their names were Scott Gilgen and Griffin Lund, and that they were fourteen years old.

"Scott and Griff," I said, "I'd like you to come in and meet my daughter."

They grinned at each other and looked nervous, I think because they assumed I had a daughter about their age. When I took them into Charity's room and introduced them to her, they were absolutely speechless. I explained Charity's situation, told them a little about her, and asked them not only to find another jump for their machines but to idle quietly and go slowly whenever they drove past our home to visit each other.

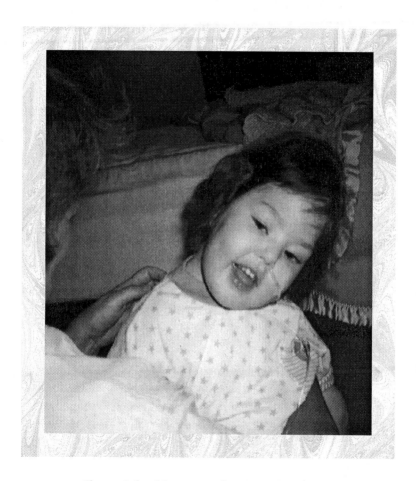

Charity's health improved in Fountain Green.

They both agreed instantly and then started asking questions about Charity. It wasn't many minutes before she had registered and accepted their voices and had begun smiling and communicating with them. From then until we left that home nearly six months later, those two young men never spoke to us without asking about Charity, and they never again jumped across our driveway or frightened her in any way with their machines.

Fountain Green is a small community, and so word of our family quickly spread. Once again, as they had in our former area, several wonderful people made themselves available for training so they could tend Charity whenever we had to leave.

Jaki Collard, one of those great helpers, wrote: "Charity was sleeping when I first saw her, and she looked like a normal, beautiful little girl. But when she awoke she was much quieter than most four-year-olds. Instead she seemed to exude a calm stillness. Her beautiful dark eyes watched everything around her, but her responses were mostly half smiles and coos—that is, until someone she knew and loved came into the room. Then she absolutely glowed. Her eyes sparkled and her smile filled the room. It was overwhelming to me."

"Once after Charity had smiled at her," wrote Cindy Anderson, another helper, "my youngest daughter, Bambi, said, 'She's an angel in disguise, isn't she.' After that, when I rocked and talked with Charity and she would smile that beautiful smile for me, I thought about what Bambi had said, and now I believe that is exactly what Charity was— an angel in disguise.

"How can I describe the feeling that was in Charity's room as well as her entire home? Never before nor since have I felt the kind of peace and serenity that I felt when I was with her. It was like a calm, sweet feeling would envelop me the moment I walked through their door. I live a very hectic life, and this was completely new for me. It was as if time stood still, a time of peace—just little Charity and myself."

Charity had been around other families than ours in her life, staying in at least three different homes on the occasions when Kathy and I had to be away for more than a day. But now a new wrinkle arose as these women ventured to bring their families into our home to be with Charity when they tended.

"Sometimes," Cindy continued, "I would come home after being with Charity and tell my husband and children about the special feeling that was with her. I knew they really didn't understand, though, so when the first opportunity came along I took them to meet her. They were totally smitten, just as I had been. My normally rowdy children became instantly quiet as they soaked in Charity's sweetness. And my family agreed with me. There was a sweet, heavenly spirit about that beautiful, happy little girl, something they could actually feel."

Jaki expressed similar feelings: "Charity had such an influence that everyone loved her and wanted to be near her. I often wondered at that, for here was a little child whom many would consider a 'throwaway baby,' an accident of birth who had no life. Yet by the power of her spirit she loved us all so deeply that we could feel it and wanted to seek after it.

"Charity didn't dance or play like other little girls. But, oh, she did do something. Something wonderful. She reminded us of the meaning of the word *love*. She influenced every life that touched hers—everyone she met and so many that she didn't meet, she loved. The spirit that she used to animate her body, in place of the brain the rest of us use, was awesome. *Is* awesome! Truly, Charity is love."

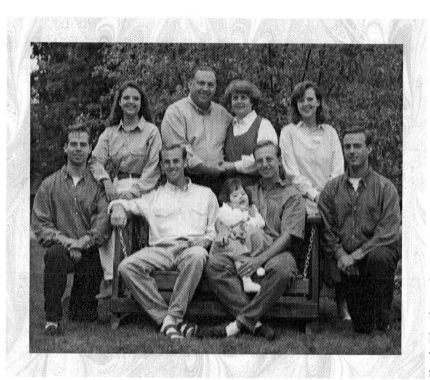

Photo by Token Photography

The Yorgason Family
Clockwise from far left: Steven, Michelle, Blaine, Kathy, Tami,
Nathan, Daniel, Charity, Travis.

YEARS OF PEACE

◆

Our first two and a half years in our new home in Salt Lake City, beginning in the fall of 1993, were amazing to both Kathy and me. Though Charity continued to have seizures and eczema and the miscellaneous other minor problems that seemed her lot in life, we hardly ever had to suction phlegm from her throat, and she completely stopped going into her down cycles of bad days. She was always alert, always happy, and always ready to impart her love to anyone willing to receive it. In short, she seemed completely at peace. Though the medical profession couldn't offer a plausible explanation for this great change, we accepted it as a wonderful blessing—for Charity and for us—and regularly gave thanks for it.

We hadn't been in our new home for more than a day or two when a very precious group of helpers put in their appearance. Upon answering the doorbell one afternoon, Kathy was surprised to see a small child looking up at her.

"I'm Alisha Earl," the child said confidently. "From across the street. Do you have any little kids I can play with?"

Welcoming her into our home, Kathy introduced Alisha to a smiling Charity, explained why Charity could not get out of bed to play, and then left them alone together. Alisha didn't stay long, ten minutes or so, but the next day she was back with her brother, Calvin, and the day after that with someone else, and soon Charity had become the hub of a group of twenty or more neighborhood children who returned again and again, sometimes singly and sometimes with others, including relatives and friends, to visit our daughter.

As time passed, these children began thinking of ways to help and entertain. Ashley Peterson and her friend made up dances to perform for Charity, while Brooke Smith and Shayla Michaels and others brought storybooks (and sometimes their mothers) and read to her, something Charity absolutely loved. She also loved the songs many of them sang for her, and she never failed to show her gratitude in the only way she could—by reaching out with her smile.

Whenever the days were warm and windless, we loaded Charity into her wheelchair and took her for walks around the neighborhood. Except for the sounds of dogs barking and jet aircraft passing overhead, she loved this, and beamed whenever we told her we were going outside. Charity was like a little Pied Piper, for we never went far before crowds of neighbor kids began gathering to her. They walked beside her, held her hands, ran their fingers through her hair, chattered quietly with us or each other or her, and simply stared in awe at this little girl who was the same as them and yet so different, so unaffected by the things of their world.

Upon moving into our new home, we also enrolled Charity in the Jordan Valley School—a school for children with assorted limitations. Though she was too fragile to attend, Charity was visited weekly in our home by physical therapists and other professionals who came to assist in her care.

The first time these women came to see Charity was an amazing experience for us. There were five or six of them, and when we took them back to meet Charity, they instantly took over. While Charity

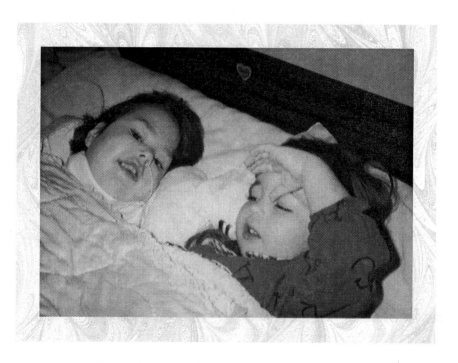

Charity having a sleep-over with her niece Jessa.

grinned from ear to ear and reveled in the attention, they lined both sides of her bed and, laughing and visiting quietly with her and each other, all went to work on her body and sundry extremities. Such unity was a surprise to me, and Kathy and I were astounded that such a busy crowd could be so tender and calming.

As she had grown older and larger, Charity's neurological damage had caused her muscles to tighten and twist, clenching her fingers, pulling her right arm and hand up against her chest and chin, twisting her left wrist and hand down and under her left arm, and wrenching both of her feet far to the right. Though Kathy and the therapists from the school worked diligently on these muscles, massaging them and working them very gently with range-of-motion therapy, after several months they determined it was not enough. Other specialists came out and created plastic splints, molded to the size and shape of Charity's arms and hands. These splints held her appendages in more appropriate positions and helped ease the pain of straining muscles. Though hard to put on because of the tightness of her muscles, these splints always brought smiles of relief from our little daughter once they were in place, and helped her relax at least temporarily.

We were also blessed by the Make-A-Wish Foundation. After several calls and visits to evaluate Charity's needs, their representatives appeared one evening with a lovely rocking love seat that was wide enough to hold both Charity and one of us without crowding. Having been told of Charity's love for music, they also brought a small stereo system that could be controlled by remote, along with several new tapes and CDs for her to listen to. The stereo, tapes, and CDs were a complete surprise to us and had not been part of Charity's wish, but were perfect for the needs of our daughter.

As in our other areas of residence, we needed to train a few neighbors to care for Charity so we could occasionally leave home together, and several of them made themselves available. Once again, Charity made deep and lasting impressions. Regrettably, it would be impossible to recount the dozens of stories shared by these people who so willingly gave of themselves to help with Charity and were in turn blessed by her radiant spirit. Person after person told us of the beautiful experiences they had had with our angel girl. Our friend Ray Brown may have summed up those feelings best: "Jesus, in the ninth chapter of John, was asked by the apostles, Who had sinned, the blind man or his parents, to have been deserving of such a fate? Jesus responded that the man's condition was not a punishment for sin, but was to be a source for the manifestation of the works of God. Hopefully each of us has met such a person, one who lets God's love shine through them. Because I felt it so clearly, I know that Charity was one such tool in God's hands, allowing him to show his love for me."

A Growing Sacrifice

"Daddy, I'm ready for my bath!"

With a sigh I hit the "save" button on my computer, stood, and walked out the door and into Charity's room. We had designed our new home with my office next to Charity's bedroom for this very purpose, so I could be immediately available whenever Kathy and Charity needed my assistance. Sometimes, however, Charity's needs failed to coincide with the mental gymnastics I seemed always in the midst of trying to perform, and it was hard to pull myself away.

"How can you get ready for a bath so quickly?" I teased as I leaned over Charity's smiling face to kiss her forehead. She responded with a kick and an even bigger grin, and feeling instantly better I kissed her again and turned to Kathy.

"Is the water in the tub?"

"Of course it is. I wouldn't have called you if it wasn't."

That made sense, but I was still amazed that I hadn't even heard the water running. Talk about a man getting into his work–

"Okay, squirt," I said, sliding one hand under Charity's neck and shoulders and the other beneath her thighs, "let's go for a ride into the bathroom."

It was a trick lifting and carrying Charity, and I was never sure that I had mastered it. Over the past two years her weight had fluctuated between 45 and 47 pounds, which isn't terribly heavy, yet she had grown steadily taller, reaching a height of about 48 inches. In all four feet she had no muscle tone whatever, but flopped about like a big rag doll whenever we moved her. So carrying her to the tub wasn't just a matter of picking her up and walking from one room to another. It meant using my left arm and hand to support her neck and head and keep them in line with her shoulders and back, positioning my upper body, neck, and chin to keep her arms and hands from dangling and banging against walls and door frames, keeping her hips straight in line with her back using my right hand, and somehow making certain that her legs and feet did not twist or get banged into anything along the way.

Charity's bones were paper-thin, decimated by osteoporosis, and broke very easily. Because one leg had broken three times and the other once, we were very concerned about hurting her. So moving her anywhere was difficult and awkward for me and quite dangerous for her. It had been nearly two years since Kathy had been able to lift her at all, let alone carry her about, so I was the designated lifter for Charity's bath as well as everything else that required her to be moved.

In the bathroom I eased to my knees and lowered Charity onto her bath chair, a specially built inclined platform made of plastic webbing and PVC pipe. This kept Charity off the bottom of the tub and elevated her head, but allowed her body to be submerged enough that she could enjoy the warmth of the water.

"There," I breathed, draping a warm, wet towel over her to keep the exposed part of her body warm, "does that feel good to you, punkin-doo?"

In response Charity beamed her pleasure and began chuckling, for except for having her hair washed she loved bathing and could not seem to get enough of the soothing warmth of the water.

As Kathy spread out the various soaps, lotions, and shampoo, I stepped back, and while she began the actual process of bathing I watched in wonder. It was a complicated procedure, arrived at through much experimentation, and it worked as well as anything we had found to keep Charity's eczema down and her skin soft and healthy and without sores. In fact, not once in her life had Charity ever developed a bedsore, during her last few years her eczema had almost always been under control, and she always smelled clean and fresh. Kathy was a remarkable caregiver, and I never stopped wondering at her intense and selfless dedication to our little daughter.

"You know," I said as Kathy busied herself with our daughter, "you are amazing. I hope you know that."

"I don't know what you're talking about."

"Your service to Charity. Hour after hour, day after day—well, I don't know how you do it."

I didn't, either. Never in my life had I imagined that an individual could so thoroughly sacrifice herself in behalf of another. Never had I supposed that such a level of service could even begin to exist. Day after grueling day, night after sleepless night, week in and week out for year after endless year I watched in awe as Kathy gave every ounce of herself and then some to our tattered little daughter. Of course, all of us did what we could to help, lifting Charity, moving her, holding and rocking her for brief periods, and helping with the rest of the work necessary to run a normal home and family. But it was my sweetheart who lived with Charity, who studied her continually, who prayed without ceasing for guidance and inspiration in her care, and who developed an uncanny sense of her needs and how best to meet them.

"Do you remember when you rented the movie *Groundhog Day?*" Kathy asked as she carefully lathered one of Charity's legs.

"Yeah," I replied with a smile, "I remember."

"Well, I had the feeling while I was watching it, especially the second time through, that the movie was really about me. When Bill Murray was watching his silly alarm clock, I knew exactly how he felt! Every day with Charity is Groundhog Day for me; every day is exactly the same. Seven days a week, fifty-two weeks a year, I wake up knowing that I am facing exactly the same tasks I faced the morning before. But where Bill Murray could change things over time, even make them better, I can't. Day after day I have to do the exact same things and still take whatever extra challenges come along."

"How do you stand it?"

Now Kathy smiled. "Love."

"You mean your love for her strengthens you?"

"I'm sure it does. And I know the Lord's love strengthens me, too. But I think the most powerful force acting on me is Charity's love. I've never felt or experienced so much love in all my life as I feel when I am with her. Though sometimes I feel totally weighed down with the burden of it, I never go into her room but what I am almost magically rejuvenated by the magnitude of her love."

I knew Kathy felt this way, and yet cracks were developing in the walls of her ability to serve, serious cracks that had me worried. Over the years of Charity's life, Kathy's back problem had grown inexplicably worse, and she was moving more and more slowly, lifting less and less, suffering intense back and leg pains both standing and sitting, and collapsing in exhaustion at every opportunity.

"The Lord is simply requiring a sacrifice of us," Kathy would respond each time I grew fretful over her condition. "This is just part of the price we must pay in return for the incredible blessings he has given us, not the least of which is the privilege of living with one of his most choice little angels."

Kathy may have been right, but that didn't stop me from worrying about her, or from feeling guilty because I wasn't somehow taking over for her with Charity. Again and again I tried to learn the minute-by-minute details of Charity's care, to place myself in Kathy's position so I could fill in better. And though I did learn to do some things that I knew helped both her and Charity, I simply did not seem able to wrap my emotions and my life around our daughter's needs the way Kathy had done. Instead, my mind just kept getting sidetracked back into my writing, as though it, rather than Kathy and Charity, were the focal point of my life.

Downhill Again

◆

In May of 1995 our son Nathan married Rachel Jones. Nate was the fifth of our six now-adult children to marry, and all five had taken this important step during Charity's lifetime. As the wedding approached, Kathy and I joked with Travis, who was not yet remotely interested in that institution, that perhaps Charity was remaining alive until all her older siblings had married. He only grinned at what he considered another feeble attempt on our part to push him toward matrimonial bliss.

During a family gathering a few days later, the subject of Charity helping Tami and Dave select each other as mates was raised, and Kathy and I began to wonder if perhaps we hadn't been joking after all.

"Tami wasn't the only one who used Charity's help," Michelle declared. "Trent and I used her too."

"How?" I asked in surprise.

Michelle smiled mischievously. "Basically, just like Tami. I could see that Charity loved Trent, which meant he was a good person. I also knew that Trent loved Charity, because he told me so. If he hadn't, I probably wouldn't have been interested in marrying him. Trent says he felt the same about me."

It turned out that to one degree or another the same was true for Dan and Rebecca, Steve and his wife, and now Nate and Rachel.

Charity had somehow influenced all of their decisions on whom to marry. Kathy and I had never heard of this, and except for Tami had not been aware that it was happening. We did know that quite often the kids had brought their dates home to meet Charity. What we hadn't realized was how profoundly they were influenced by their friends' reactions to Charity, and hers to them. Evidently none of our children could imagine marrying a person who didn't love their little sister. From what they told us that day, it seemed that more than a few had failed and were no longer dated. But of the ones who passed and went on to become our children-in-law, Kathy and I had often remarked that we could not have selected better ourselves.

As their wedding approached, Nate and Rachel decided that our home would be a nice place for their open house. Kathy and I quickly agreed, thinking that Charity's room was far enough away from where the guests would be that she would be protected from the noise. As added insurance, we asked our friend Ann Mickelsen to come sit with her, to keep the door closed as much as possible, and to keep Charity's visitors (especially our growing brood of grandchildren) quiet and under control.

The open house went well, and Nate and Rachel were pleased to visit with those who came to honor them. As the evening was concluding, however, Ann stepped out to inform us that Charity was not doing well at all. Far more guests than we had anticipated had wanted to greet Charity, her door had constantly been opened and closed, some had kept their voices low while others had not, and Ann had finally placed a big note on the door stating that Charity had gone to sleep.

Unfortunately, she was not asleep when we got back to her, but was trembling and whimpering and looking for all the world like she was

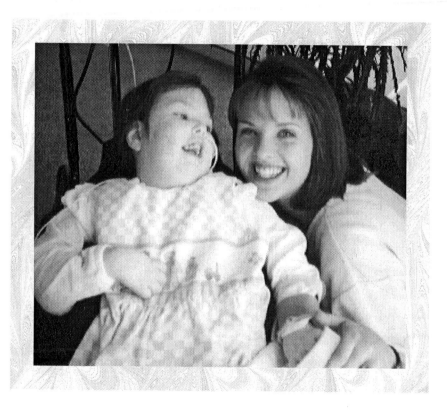

Charity and Michelle share a smile together.

going into a dive caused by head pressures—something we had not seen in nearly three years.

For a day or so we clung to the hope that Charity's struggles were merely a reaction to the noise and confusion, but it was soon evident that they were not. Her cycles of pressure had returned, though not as severely or frequently as before. But the occasional down times were definitely one more thing Kathy had to deal with each day—one more burden to place atop her almost unbearable load.

A NEW BOOK

"Blaine, you received a letter from Karen Boren at the *Deseret News*."

Looking up from my computer keyboard, where I was doing my typical, three-fingered best, I took the letter and tore it open.

"I hope she isn't trying to talk us into doing a newspaper article on Charity again." Kathy sounded exhausted and worried. "I just think that kind of notoriety would put too much stress in her life. Didn't we explain that to Karen, Blaine?"

"We did," I mumbled while I tried to read. "Last year, when she came out with some of her family to meet Charity. And at least once on the telephone since then."

Kathy sighed. "I hope she understands."

"Kath," I said, looking up from the single page Karen had sent me, "that isn't what this is about."

"What is it, then?" Kathy was obviously relieved.

Slowly I shook my head. "This is an Associated Press news release, written by somebody named Lindsey Tanner and put out through the *New York Times* News Service on 24 May 1995. It says that between 1,000 and 2,000 U.S. infants are born each year with anencephaly, in which most or all of the brain, and sometimes portions of the skull and scalp, are missing, leaving them without life or consciousness."

"Makes you wonder how such smart people can be so stupid," Kathy grumbled uncharacteristically. "Without life or consciousness? Good grief! They need to come and meet Charity."

I grinned. "It would help, but only if they could get past her mother. Listen to the rest of this. 'Fewer than half survive more than a day, and more than 90 percent are dead within a week. Their vital organs deteriorate as they slip toward death, rendering them useless for transplants unless removed soon after birth.'"

"Transplants?"

"That's right," I said as I quickly read on down. "Did you catch that? They want to remove their organs soon after birth. They call it 'harvesting.' The American Medical Association's Council on Ethical and Judicial Affairs, a nine-member committee whose opinions are considered AMA policy, have called for the legal right to remove organs from such children when they are newly born but still living, to be donated out to others."

Kathy looked at me, her expression puzzled. "I don't understand. How can they remove organs from living babies without . . . without—?"

Soberly I nodded. "That's right, hon. What this AMA Council on Ethical and Judicial Affairs wants is the legal right to kill babies like Charity so they can 'harvest' the organs and transplant them to others."

"But . . . but that's *murder!*"

I nodded my agreement. "And isn't 'harvesting' a nice-sounding word for it? Makes them sound like benevolent farmers. This is incredible!"

"Well, somebody ought to tell them about babies like Charity."

"Yeah," I responded, "that's what Karen says, here in the margin.

Somebody ought to tell them, and she thinks it should be us. She thinks it's time we wrote a book about our experiences with Charity."

It was the beginning of June, 1995. Charity's pressure had once again diminished, and she was back to enjoying a great deal of peace. Nevertheless, she was getting more fragile, more frightened by noise, more in need of a very quiet and peaceful environment. She still enjoyed visitors, but we were now forced to limit them to one or two at a time, especially if they intended to stay longer than a minute or so. Otherwise the babble of voices proved too much for Charity to deal with, and she would become distressed and burst into tears.

This is what we had explained to Karen some time before, when we had been introduced by mutual friends and she had brought some of her family to meet Charity. She felt that Charity's story would make a wonderful feature for her paper, but we feared that the publicity would simply bring too many people to our door and increase the stress on our fragile little daughter. Hence we had declined any sort of article concerning Charity.

I did not immediately respond to Karen about the press release, but I saved it, and off and on for the next few weeks I thought about it, wondering if I really should write a book about Charity.

Early in August a longtime friend, Stewart Beveridge, stopped by to see me. I had run into him a few weeks earlier and told him a little about Charity, and he had wanted to meet her. She was gracious as usual when I introduced them, filled with her special brand of joy, and within a few seconds she had completely captured Stew's heart. In fact, as he was leaving our home he showed me his arms, covered with goose bumps, and told me he had never felt so overwhelmed. A week later he was back with his wife, Gaye, and a week after that he called to make another appointment to see me.

Sitting in my office that afternoon in late August, Stew came right to the point. "Blaine," he declared, "in my opinion Charity's story is the most incredible thing I have ever heard, and I believe it should be shared with the world. If you will write it, my friend Craig Middleton and I would like to publish it."

To my amazement, as Stew said this I felt very strongly that he was right. It was indeed time to write my angel's story. More than that, as I sat facing Stew the story actually unfolded in my mind, so that in less time than I am taking now to write this sentence I could envision the entire format of the book.

Because of the position taken by the AMA, it seemed that it was time for Kathy, Charity, and me to make a stand—to declare before the world that anencephalic and hydranencephalic children did indeed live and have consciousness. More important, I felt that I needed to tell the world that Charity and other children with limitations, no matter the extent, were beloved of God as choice individual beings, and could make incredibly positive contributions to homes and families. I knew, for our family had been so blessed.

By that evening I was hard at work, and three months later the first copy of Charity's story (the first sixteen months of her life) rolled off the presses. During that time I had had several additional conversations with Karen Boren, and finally we had agreed that she could bring a news photographer into our home and do a feature story.

The original version of *One Tattered Angel,* a small paperback edition, first hit the stores on December 1, 1995, and Karen's story, covering both our life with Charity and the AMA's resolution concerning the harvesting of organs, was set to run in the *Deseret News* on

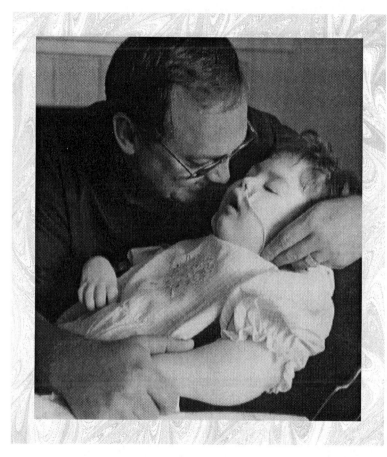

Photo by Kristan Jacobsen, Deseret News

This picture of Blaine and Charity appeared
in the Deseret News *article.*

December 6. Interestingly, on December 5, before they had ever even seen the book, the AMA's Council on Ethical and Judicial Affairs decided to table their resolution about taking organs from living anencephalic donors until it could be studied more thoroughly. Karen was able to learn of this new development, do some quick telephone interviews, and make the AMA's new official position a sidebar to her story about Charity:

AMA SUSPENDS RECOMMENDATION ON ANENCEPHALIC BABIES

In a telephone call from Washington, D.C., on Tuesday, Dr. Charles Plows, chairman of the American Medical Association's Council on Ethical and Judicial Affairs, told the *Deseret News,* 'We are suspending the (May 1995) action of the council until we get more input one way or the other on the level of consciousness in these neonates (newborns) . . . '

Dr. Marion L. Walker, director of pediatric neurosurgery at Primary Children's Medical Center, is also relieved this policy has been suspended. 'American physicians aren't ready to start taking the lives of babies,' he said.

Local public response to both the news article and our book was overwhelming. Letters started pouring in, requests to meet Charity were declined as politely as possible, and wherever Kathy or I went, people wanted to talk about our daughter. Most surprising to me were the numbers of people who also had or at least knew angelically gifted children. People and families everywhere, even though many had not thought in such terms until they had read Charity's story, were being blessed in ways very similar to ours.

A couple of months later, when two local television stations decided to do stories about her, we could see that Charity's influence was indeed spreading. As we watched Channel 5 News reporters Shelley Osterloh and Carol Mikita, and a few weeks later Fox 13 News reporter Shauna Parsons, report their findings, we both felt a growing sense of awe.

Who was this child? we continued to wonder. And how in the world had we been so fortunate as to have been made a part of her life?

PREMONITIONS AND DREAMS

◆───

   "What will we do, Blaine, when I no longer have the strength to care for Charity?"

"Do you really think it will come to that?"

Kathy sighed. "The way I feel, it's coming to that very quickly."

For a few moments I stared up into the darkness. "I know I haven't been able to do this yet, Kath, but I'm certain I could learn all the little things you do, and just take over."

"You already do a lot, honey, but you could never become her mother. That's me. The Lord has blessed me with an ongoing sense of her needs that no one else could possibly have, you included. Besides, if you started spending full time with Charity, who would earn the living around here?"

"I could show you how to write," I stated seriously.

"Sure!" Kathy sighed. "Honestly, Blaine, we might have to think about an institution for Charity."

"Could you do that?" I asked gently.

Silently my sweetheart shook her head, and I could tell that she was suddenly weeping. "I . . . I couldn't stand it!"

"Neither could I," I responded, climbing out of bed. "I'd stop writing before it ever came to that!"

It was the week before Christmas, 1995, and still dark as I pulled out of the driveway to attend a series of book signings for *One Tattered Angel* in a couple of distant communities. I drove mechanically, preoccupied with the issues I was struggling with and hoping for some resolution. Something had to happen, I knew that—and soon. Not only was life getting more difficult for Charity, but Kathy's health was also deteriorating rapidly, and I didn't think she would be able to hold up much longer either.

Meanwhile, I continued to be unable to offer more than what I considered to be superficial help to the two of them. I fretted so much about this that my worries probably contributed significantly to the problem. I know for a fact that they took some of the joy out of my interaction with Kathy and Charity.

During the course of that December day, I found myself offering up quick mental prayers every time I got back in my car to change locations. I don't know exactly what I was hoping for. I think mainly I just wanted to remind the Lord that we were in the midst of a serious problem, and to ask for whatever help he thought might be appropriate. What happened during my drive home, therefore, came as a complete surprise, and it left me stunned.

As if from nowhere these words appeared in my consciousness: *Prepare your mind, for your daughter is about to depart from you.* Startled, I tried to think around them, if that makes any sense. But no matter what I did or tried to think about, the words would not go away. Again and again they seemed to be repeated: *Prepare your mind, for your daughter is about to depart from you.*

At home that evening I told Kathy of my experience and asked if she had felt anything similar. She replied that she had not, and together we sat and worried about precisely what it meant. We didn't doubt it, at least not exactly. It was just that Charity's heart seemed so strong, and she had overcome so many impossible odds in her seven and a half years, that neither of us could imagine that my premonition could possibly be correct.

However, several times during the next few months I "heard" in my mind the same edict. Sometimes the words seemed to vary slightly, but never the message. It was always the same. It seemed that we needed to get prepared, for the Lord was getting ready to call our little darling home.

The thing was, we had no idea of how to prepare, or of when Charity might pass away. From the day we had discovered the terrible extent of her disabilities, we had been anticipating her death. If anything, after nearly eight years we felt less prepared for it than ever. Our lives had become so entwined together, and there was such great joy in our home and in our family because of her, that we could not even imagine a life without our beloved little Charity. Every time we talked about it we ended up in tears, and neither of us could begin to comprehend how we would ever cope with such a loss.

One morning in April 1996, we received a phone call from our daughter Tami, who was living at that time in Fort Dodge, Iowa.

"Mom and Dad," she said as she fought to keep her emotions under control, "I . . . I think Charity is going to pass away—very soon."

"Why?" I asked, immediately thinking of the feelings I had been having.

"You know how I've always wanted to write a song for her, but couldn't? Well, my impression has been that no song would come until she died. Only then would the Lord give me a song for her."

"And it came?" Kathy asked almost fearfully.

"It . . . started to. This morning. For some reason I had been thinking about Charity ever since I awoke, and a little while ago the song suddenly started filling my mind."

"Oh, Tami . . ."

"Mom, it is absolutely beautiful! I've called it 'I Believe in Angels.' The music is so clear in my mind that I can play it perfectly. Both hands. The thing is, I don't have all the words yet. I have the first part, but not the rest of it."

"Have you written it down?" I asked.

"I've written the words so far, but I haven't written the music because I don't know enough theory to do that correctly."

"What happens if you forget it?"

I could hear Tami smiling through her tears. "Dad, if this is a song the Lord wants me to sing for Charity, he won't let me forget it. Only," and now her voice broke again, "I can't stand the thought of . . . of losing my little Chare-bear . . ."

A day or so after Tami's call, our friends Ken and Brenda Gallacher dropped by. We had not spent much time with them in recent months, so for a few minutes we visited, catching up on each other's lives.

"Well," Ken finally said, looking awfully reluctant, "I mentioned to Kathy last week when I bumped into her that I had had a dream about Charity."

I nodded. "She told me that. Are you going to tell us the dream?"

"I think so." Ken grinned teasingly. "No, I am. I haven't wanted to, I can tell you that. But if it turns out that the dream is real and I didn't tell you—well, I'd feel awful."

For a moment nobody spoke, nobody stirred.

"I don't know why I'm having a dream about Charity, either," Ken abruptly continued. "I'm not a close relative, or anyone special who has known your family for any great length of time. I'm only someone you've had to tolerate for a couple of years as a neighbor, which for you has probably been long enough."

Ken grinned and we chuckled with him.

"Anyway," he said, suddenly serious again, "I have been very humbled by this. I just hope you find it helpful."

Then, drawing a deep breath, Ken began to speak. "In the early hours of one morning back in February or March, I had this unusual dream. It wasn't the ordinary type of dream where logic is somehow distorted; I could feel the thoughts and communications of the individuals I saw without verbal communication. The sensations I felt were strong and realistic."

Ken went on to describe in great detail how he had seen Charity being cared for by a baby-sitter who was distressed because she thought she had done something to cause Charity to suffer. Kathy and I apparently came home from a lengthy trip at that moment, and we were trying to reassure the sitter and at the same time care for our daughter, when she suddenly began to die. Apparently we realized this, and felt peaceful about it. Shortly afterward two radiant women descended into the room in a beam or conduit of light. One of them reached out and motioned toward Charity's still form, and an extraordinarily beautiful young woman rose up from where she lay. Though she appeared much older than Charity, it was clear to Ken that this lovely young woman was her. Charity then followed the two women up the beam of light, but not before stopping and, in a glorious but indescribable manifestation, communicating her love to Kathy and me one final time.

"I was jolted awake at that moment," Ken said, "and looked at my clock on the nightstand. It was 3:00 A.M. I awoke Brenda and asked her if she had felt anything, and then I related the experience I had just dreamt. Later I sat at my desk for a long time, wondering why in the world I would be privy to such an event. I knew it was no ordinary dream, so I just kept asking myself: 'Why?' As I said, I have been really struggling with this, as I felt such sensitivity for you both. Still, knowing that I would regret not having told you should Charity pass away very soon, Brenda and I decided that tonight would be a good time to share.

"I want you to know that I have felt ever since the dream that it was a sacred, special event that rightfully belongs to the two of you. There is no way to justify or prove what I saw, but I will never deny what I felt—an absolutely incredible amount of love."

A Sweet Message

"Hi, hon." I was still buttoning my shirt as I walked into Charity's room. "Morning, Punkin-doo. How come you two got up so early?"

Both Kathy and Charity smiled. "This is one of Charity's party days, Daddy. She was awake by 4:00, wanting to talk to me, so I turned off the monitor and let you sleep."

"You wanted to talk to Mommy?" I teased as I nuzzled and kissed our beaming little angel. It was May, 1996, she was closing in on eight years of age now, and to me she was the most beautiful little girl in the world. I could never seem to get enough of just looking at her. "Well, squirt, when are you going to talk to me?"

At that Charity burst into her delightful, deep-voiced chuckle. I kissed her a few more times, and looked back at Kathy. "You really have been talking with her?" I asked.

"I've had some interesting feelings this morning," Kathy responded as she tugged on Charity's socks. "About you."

"Me?"

"You know how people are always telling us how they can feel Charity's thoughts and desires? Well, this morning when I was changing her, I had the strongest impression that Charity wanted me to tell you something." My wife smiled and pulled a sticky note off the love seat. "This is it. If Charity could talk, I believe this is what she would say to you. The handwriting, of course, is mine."

Taking the note I sat down, and while Charity snorted the way she did when she got excited, and then began chuckling again, I read: *"Daddy, please stop worrying and start being happy. You can't take care of my physical needs the way Mom does, but she can't be my spokesman, my voice. Only you can tell the world who I am, what I think, and how I feel. I am so pleased that you are willing to be open enough to do so. Together you and Mom are making my life more wonderful than I ever thought possible.*

"Remember, Daddy, I love you more than you can know—"

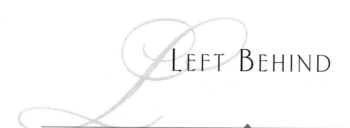

LEFT BEHIND

"Are you nervous about going home?" I asked.

It was the second day of June, 1996, and we were just coming out of the canyon and back into the Salt Lake Valley.

"You mean, finding out if something has happened to Charity while we've been away?"

"Uh-huh, just like Ken dreamed."

For a moment Kathy looked away from the freeway and into the distance. "A little," she finally responded. "But it's more than Ken's dream, Blaine, a lot more. Besides your feelings and Tami's, I worry about the way Charity has been struggling. I don't know what happened to her the night of Nate's open house last year, but since then she's had a pretty difficult time of it."

"You mean her head pressures?"

"Well, it was head pressure up until three or four weeks ago." Kathy leaned back and closed her eyes. "At first I thought it was pressure this time too. But her eyes haven't constricted, so I don't know. She's been so erratic lately. I just wish I knew what was going on."

"And I wish her giggles would come back," I added. "This past month, ever since her little one-day party, it's been hard for her to even work up a smile."

"I know, Blaine. I miss them too. What really worries me, though, is that I don't think her poor little body can stand much more of this. I know I don't want her to suffer any longer—not if it means going through this type of ordeal all the time. It just isn't fair."

I was as worried as Kathy. In fact, both of us had called home more often than we usually did, trying somehow to put off what we both felt was inevitable. Ken, as he had related his dream, could not have known that for the first time in years I had agreed the previous fall to several two- or three-day book-signing and speaking trips during the coming spring, one of which had included Kathy. We had also scheduled a quick springtime trip to see Tami and David and their children. Of course, since Ken and Brenda's visit we had asked each other the same thing every time we went anywhere together, even when we had left Charity with one of our well-trained and experienced baby-sitters.

As it turned out, upon our return that day we discovered that something *had* happened. One of the caregivers, in lifting or rolling Charity to change a diaper or something, had apparently forgotten (or not understood) how fragile her little body was. Charity was stressed and agitated, and each time we moved her legs or hips, her eyes went wide with fear and she whimpered in pain. That was not a good sign.

In consultation with Dr. Schmidt, however, we concluded to delay the ambulance ride (which terrified Charity, but was the only way we dared take her to the doctor anymore) and see if the problem would work itself out. In fact, we weren't even sure what or where the problem was—a broken bone or merely a pulled or strained muscle somewhere in her back, hips, or legs. Within a few days Charity seemed to be doing better, and so we never did take her in for X-rays or an examination.

As we moved through the first three weeks of June, Charity continued her ups and downs. She had never been a spitty child, and had gone years without throwing up. But several times in those three weeks she threw up for no reason that we could see. The odd thing was, she usually smiled afterward, as if to say that she felt better and that we didn't need to worry. Yet whenever I thought about it, something continued to whisper quietly, *Prepare your mind, for your daughter is about to depart from you.*

On Saturday, June 22, 1996, Charity awakened us a little before 4:00 A.M. with more of her giggles. On hurrying into her room, we were thrilled to see once again the joy in her countenance. It was as if her bad days were all behind her, and only happiness stretched ahead.

Charity smiled and laughed and carried on with us and with whoever else came near all that day. Even with a sedative she didn't sleep much Saturday night, and her personal party continued throughout Sunday. It was wonderful to behold. Some of our children and grandchildren came by and joined in the revelry, and it was a delightful time for all of us.

The laughing and smiles continued on Monday, and now Kathy and I were beginning to wonder. What could have happened to bring about such an amazing change? Neither of us knew, of course, but we were so thrilled that Charity was feeling well and was back to her smiles and laughter that we refused to worry about it. I even took a few photographs Monday afternoon, feeling an urgency to preserve such expressive and radiant joy.

Looking back now, I am dumbfounded that neither Kathy nor I understood the significance of Charity's joy. Just as she had rejoiced and thrown a personal party in the hospital the night the doctors had removed her final shunt and prepared her to return home with us, we now understand that she was doing the same thing again. For seven years and ten months she had successfully taught and blessed the lives

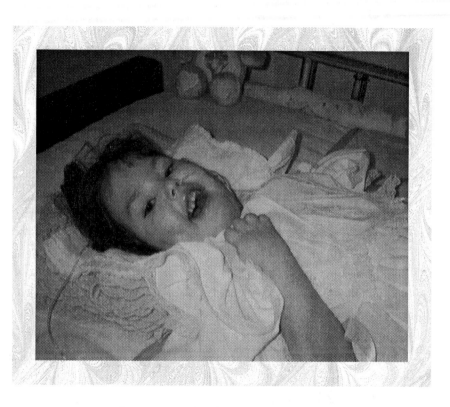

Charity never lost her contagious smile.

of her family and countless others, spreading happiness and love to all who would receive it, and at last she was finished. With incredible courage she had run her mortal race, passed the test of physical pain and suffering, and endured to the end. She knew this! She knew, too, that the Lord had done all he could to prepare us for her departure. I don't think she knew how much we would sorrow and grieve—how terribly we would miss her. But I don't think she was supposed to know that. Had she known, she might have tried to stay, and in the eternal scheme of things we know that would not have been right.

Anyway, at about 10:00 Monday night, while she was still smiling and laughing with the sheer joy of her angelic accomplishments, I wheeled Charity into her room and lifted her into bed. She gave me her typical, huge, "thank-you" smile, I kissed her forehead and gently rubbed the front of her thigh (which she dearly loved—perhaps because of the previous fractures and bony growth in that spot), and then Kathy took over and began the process of getting her ready for bed.

Fifteen minutes later, Charity suddenly began throwing up, over and over in a manner such as we had never seen her do, and all through the night we were kept busy cleaning up and trying to comfort her. And trying to comfort ourselves, too, for in the bile she vomited at the last we saw what we thought might be blood. Neither of us knew exactly what this meant, but we knew it could not be anything good, and so our worries grew worse.

At about 3:00 A.M. Charity's heaving finally eased and she drifted into a comatose state. For the rest of the night Kathy stayed in her room while I lay listening to her breathing over the monitor and staring into the darkness, sick with worry over what was happening to our daughter.

Early Tuesday morning Kathy called Charity's doctor, who felt she most likely had a virus or the flu. He also said a small amount of blood was normal in the bile of people with dry heaves, and that the end of Charity's NG tube could easily have scratched her stomach lining when it was convulsing. Somewhat relieved, we cleaned Charity up, put her on Pedialite instead of her formula because she was still occasionally heaving, and discussed the fact that her breathing was becoming more labored—that, and her diaper that morning had been dry. We didn't know exactly what these things meant, but we did know that with the exception of the spinal meningitis we had never seen our little daughter so ill.

Throughout the day Charity's condition continued to deteriorate. Her breathing grew more labored, her diaper remained almost totally dry, and she was definitely comatose. Certainly Charity had been sick before in her life, but somehow she had always managed to pull out of it. Despite her serious symptoms, for some reason Kathy and I fully expected that she would do the same thing again. Neither of us even thought that she might truly be close to death. In fact, as I spoke on the telephone with each of our children Tuesday afternoon, telling them what was happening with Charity, I felt no sense of urgency at all. Virtually every one of us was certain she would recover.

Late Tuesday night our friend Chad Campbell, who was also a local church leader, dropped in to see how Charity was doing. He wrote: "Blaine had called and told me of Charity's illness, but it was a terribly hectic night for me. I had several people to see, and it was quite late when I finished. As I stopped at an intersection near the Yorgasons' home I had the distinct impression that I needed to go there—right then.

"Kathy was leaving as I drove up, I think to get some medication, and she invited me to open the door and walk in. I did, and found Blaine in Charity's room with big tears in his eyes because little Charity was in so much pain.

"Reaching down I took her hand, as I had always done, and began to caress it. Blaine stopped me, telling me it caused her too much pain. But then she broke into a sweet smile, and both of us knew that it didn't hurt her and that she wanted me to continue. 'Would you look at that?' Blaine said. 'She's been in so much pain that she hasn't smiled in days!'

"With Blaine I laid my hands on Charity's sweet little head. I remember looking at her just before my prayer and noticing that her eyes were watching me, taking in every movement. I don't remember what I said as we blessed her, but I remember Charity was peaceful and contented, and I knew she would soon be returning to her Father in Heaven. I felt so honored and spiritually blessed to be there, to be praying over a pure little soul who would soon be standing with God in her full natural self rather than her handicapped little body. I know this is so, and testify to it. How great my joy will be when this life is over and I will have the opportunity of meeting her again and walking and talking with her, for, from the instant we met, Charity and I have been true friends."

Chad Campbell's blessing comforted Kathy and me greatly. But by 1:30 Wednesday morning Charity's breathing had grown raspy and terribly labored, and whatever comfort we had felt earlier was gone. As she gasped for every breath, she appeared so miserable that Kathy threw herself into my arms, sobbing with helplessness. Not even with her meningitis years before had Charity suffered so terribly, and both of us were completely distraught.

"Oh, babydoll," Kathy sobbed as she caressed Charity's cheeks and tried in vain to comfort her, "please don't be sick like this. Mommy can't bear to see you suffering so."

Even though it was the middle of the night, when she was in better control of herself Kathy called Dr. Schmidt again, just as he had instructed earlier. After listening to Charity's breathing over the telephone, he recommended a slight change in her medication and suggested that we sit her up in her wheelchair. Those things did help, and for the rest of the night Kathy and I took turns in the easy chair beside Charity while she slept.

Later that morning Dr. Schmidt called to see how Charity was doing, and he sent two nurses to draw blood and do what they could to help us with Charity. By noon we could see that it wasn't turning out to be a very good day for any of us. The nurses had had a difficult time finding Charity's veins, the new NG tube hadn't gone in for them, and all the while Charity's breathing had continued to be very labored. When one of them finally called Dr. Schmidt to report this, he immediately sent out a respiratory therapist, who found Charity's blood oxygen level at 63 instead of the 90+ it should have been. Quickly Charity was placed on oxygen, and everyone seemed to breathe a sigh of relief.

By now it was late afternoon, and people had been coming and going all day, not just for Charity but with issues pertaining to my writing. Michelle had even driven in from Idaho with her baby, Hailey, because she felt like she wanted to help us during Charity's illness. And I had hardly had time to do much more than pop in and out of Charity's room. It was a crazy day, and I wasn't there to hear the respiratory therapist tell Kathy that, even with oxygen, Charity's blood oxygen level had now dropped to 52.

"This oxygen isn't doing her any good," the therapist declared as she adjusted the dials and took additional readings.

"What would you do if she was your little girl?" Kathy pleaded desperately.

"If she was my little girl," the woman responded quietly, "I'd cry."

As Kathy tearfully told me this a few moments later, both of us finally realized that Charity was dying, though we had no idea how soon she would go. In fact, as each of our children had called during the day I had once again calmed their fears, telling them I was certain there was no urgency in coming to Charity's side. Now, as I hurriedly tried to call them back, I could find none of them. Even Travis, who had been worried enough to stay around home nearly all day, had gone to work once Charity had been put on oxygen. Like the rest of us, he had seen her rally so often that he fully expected her to pull it off once again.

At around 5:00 in the afternoon our friends Jim and Ann Mickelsen dropped by. Together Jim and I gave Charity another blessing, her second in two days, and afterward she relaxed. I felt then that she was dying immediately, not in another day or so, and suddenly it seemed like my heart was going to break. I couldn't imagine what I would do without my little punkin-doo and her perfect, radiant love. I couldn't imagine how I would even live! Besides, what would our wonderfully accepting children do without Charity's heavenly love and influence in their lives or in the lives of their own children? And oh, what would my poor sweetheart do without the precious, minute-by-minute companionship of her beloved little Chare-bear?

After Jim and Ann had said their good-byes and gone, Kathy and Michelle sat weeping on Charity's love seat. Drying my own eyes and steeling myself as best I could against what I knew was coming, I carefully disconnected all of Charity's tubes and gadgets, lifted her, and laid her across both Michelle's and Kathy's laps. Finally I knelt in front of all of them and gently took hold of Charity's little hand. Tearfully we watched as our angel daughter, now at peace, began slipping away.

"This is so final," Kathy whispered as her tears fell unheeded. "I . . . I don't know if I can stand it!"

Reaching over, Michelle caressed her mother's hand, trying to take comfort as well as to give it. With her other hand she had been tenderly rubbing Charity's soft little feet.

"There are so many things I want to say to her," Kathy continued, "but now I . . . I can't think of any of them. Oh, my sweet little baby-doll! I am so happy for you—so thankful that you are finally at peace! I hope you know how much I have loved you. Please don't ever forget me—"

"She won't, Mom," Michelle whispered brokenly. "She won't ever forget any of us!"

At a little after 6:00 P.M. I was suddenly overwhelmed with the feeling that a door had opened somewhere and Charity's room had filled with people—individuals from the world of spirits. I didn't actually see or hear anything, but the feeling was so strong that I cannot begin to describe it. Neither can I describe the excitement that was in the air. It was as though hundreds of people had come crowding into that tiny room of Charity's, all of them bursting with excitement to greet this glorious being who had for so long been away from them, imprisoned within her tattered mortal body.

The intensity of this feeling continued to increase even as Charity's breathing grew more shallow, more slow. Then, somehow (and I can no more explain this than our friends and family could ever explain how Charity made them feel better about things) I "knew" that the two glorious, angelic women Ken Gallacher had seen in his dream had descended and were now standing above us, beckoning Charity to arise.

An instant later she opened her eyes and looked directly up at Kathy, as if she wanted to say *'Thank you'* to her dear and loving mother one last time. Then our beloved angel closed her eyes again, sighed softly as her body relaxed, and was free.

It was 6:25 P.M., June 26, 1996. And as suddenly as that, we were left alone.

A POTPOURRI OF MIRACLES

◆

Following Charity's death, which we later learned had come about because her brain stem had simply worn out, shutting her organs down one at a time, I was dumbfounded at the depth of my grief and loneliness. I had expected there to be some sort of relief because certain pressures were eased, but there was none. I had also supposed, because of the understanding I had developed of Charity's eternal nature, as well as my slowly increasing faith in the Lord Jesus Christ and his redemption, that my pain and sorrow would somehow be eliminated and I would feel only joy.

I didn't. In the days and weeks following Charity's passing I experienced such incredible sorrow and loneliness that I became almost incapable of doing anything but grieving. Practically every waking thought centered on the fact that our little darling was gone. I couldn't work. I couldn't step out of my office without turning automatically toward her bedroom—and having the emptiness of it slam me in the face. I couldn't look at Kathy without both of us bursting into tears. Charity's mortal life had ended, she had left us behind, and never again in my lifetime would I have the joy of seeing her beautiful smile, hearing her giggle, or holding her close while I sang my silly little love songs and partook of her glorious love.

Worse, though—far worse—were the pain and loneliness Kathy was suffering. I thought, having lived and worked in the same home with my sweetheart through the years, that I had understood a little about the depths of a mother's love. But as I watched her in the days, weeks, and months following Charity's death, listened to her pour out her heart to God in supplication for peace, and saw the anguish that filled her eyes and her countenance day after day, I came to understand that in many ways she and Charity had become one. Because of Charity's great and constant needs, as well as Kathy's perfect willingness to give her all in service, mother and daughter had somehow become extensions of each other. With Charity's passing, part of Kathy had also died, and I didn't know if she would ever recover.

Apparently she had the same worries concerning me.

However, God has interesting ways of showing his suffering children that he is still God. He continues to part small and personal Red Seas so that those who try in their own meager ways to love and honor him might not drown but pass through their trials on dry ground.

So it was with us. Almost immediately after Charity's death a series of small miracles began occurring. Rather than detailing all of them, I will share a few specific experiences that allowed us to know that God still loved us and that Charity had not gone far, but was still very much involved in our lives.

Almost from the day Charity came into our lives, I had worried about writing her obituary. I don't know why this troubled me so, but it did. My worries had grown after she had contracted spinal meningitis, for despite the gravity of her illness I had been unable to write anything that sounded remotely worthy of her. I mean, I had worked on that thing for days and days, and had never even managed a satisfactory rough draft.

The night of Charity's passing I awoke with a start while it was still dark, the words of her obituary clear in my mind. I arose, went into my office, and in about fifteen minutes wrote it all down. In the morning I showed Kathy the page I had written. She read it and without any hesitation (this is something my wife *never* does) told me I had forgotten a paragraph that needed to be inserted. Immediately I knew she was right. It took perhaps five additional minutes to correct my error, and the obituary was completed.

With the exception of information on survivors and the funeral, and though the published versions varied slightly from paper to paper, it was written as follows:

CHARITY AFTON YORGASON

Our beloved Tattered Angel Charity returned to her heavenly home on June 26, 1996. There she greeted the hosts on high, who have for so long missed her joyful presence.

Born August 30, 1988, Charity came with less than almost any other mortal. Yet her desire was to serve the Lord Jesus Christ, and so within hours she began giving of her heart, her very soul, to all who came near. With her bright and dancing eyes, her smile that lit the darkest of rooms and days, her serenity-filled spirit, and her body-shaking chuckle that acknowledged a joy that never for a moment diminished, she faced life squarely. Without ever speaking a word she taught of faith, of hope, of compassion, of courage, of patience, and especially of love. And when we and others despaired of her life because it did not seem possible for her to endure or continue, she merely smiled—and did.

Yet not alone did she travel, for there are many who have served her along the way—kind and tender-hearted individuals who have given of themselves to her when it was neither easy nor convenient. These—doctors, nurses, therapists, family, friends, neighbors, and especially the children who loved to drop in and visit—all these have our eternal gratitude, and we know that Charity will bless their names forever.

And so now she has finished the course God set for her, and with lightened heart has gone ahead, to be encircled about eternally in the arms of Christ's love.

Charity, each of us knows that we will see you again soon. And though you will be perfected and given all that you have lacked and more, you will never be more precious or dear than you have been while angelically gracing our earthly home.

We were overwhelmed by the wonderful response of people to both Charity's wake, or viewing, and her funeral service, where we had the privilege of greeting friends, loved ones, and kindhearted strangers who came to pay their final respects to our daughter. Yet my entire family dreaded these events as we went into them, for we knew the terrible toll that standing in one place for more than a few minutes at a time took upon Kathy's health. It had been two or three years since she had been able to stand still without suffering untold agony, and so our children and I were all worried.

As the viewing moved through its nearly five hours of uninterrupted greeting, every one of us offered Kathy chairs, a stool, a few moments to lie down—anything to ease her burden. To our surprise, she turned us down and continued standing and reaching out to the people who had loved our daughter.

Much later that night, as we were riding home, Kathy expressed her amazement that she had felt no pain or fatigue. It had been, she tried to explain, almost as though someone had been standing behind her with their arms around her, lifting her so that her own body had no weight whatsoever.

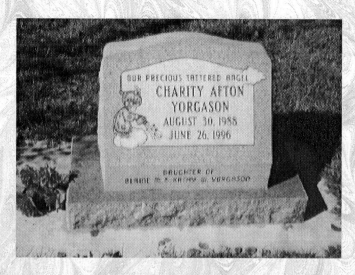

OUR PRECIOUS TATTERED ANGEL
CHARITY AFTON
YORGASON
AUGUST 30, 1988
JUNE 26, 1996

DAUGHTER OF
BLAINE M. & KATHY W. YORGASON

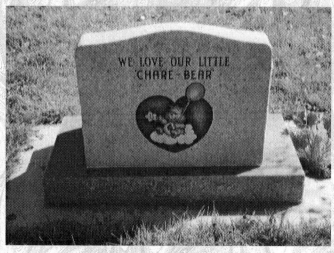

WE LOVE OUR LITTLE
'CHARE-BEAR'

This miracle continued the next day as she stood greeting people for another couple of hours, then stood again at the podium and spoke movingly of her angel daughter and the exquisite love they had shared. It went on all the remainder of the day, so that not once in that twenty-four-hour period did Kathy experience any physical pain or exhaustion.

To be truthful, both of us wondered if she had somehow been healed. We certainly hoped for it. Sadly, that notion was dispelled the day after the funeral when Kathy's body returned to its more normal, more painful, behavior. Though I suppose what happened is open to a certain amount of speculation, Kathy is convinced that she was lifted and sustained by the arms and love of a precious, grateful daughter.

Another little miracle that touched our hearts was the conclusion of our daughter Tami's episode with the song she was writing about Charity. After her call to us, she continued to play the song over and over, day after day, fearing and yet knowing that this song was being given to her as a final tribute to her beloved little sister. Then came our two or three calls about Charity's illness and the announcement of her passing. Tami was left desolate. Again she sat at her piano, and this time the final verse came to her.

As a result of several generous offers, Tami was able to record the music, and a few days later we were all edified as she sang "her" song at Charity's funeral. Those words, which she has now copyrighted, are as follows:

> *I BELIEVE IN ANGELS*
>
> *Every now and then when I see you*
> *I see heaven.*
> *Every now and then when I hold you close*
> *I feel a little of forever.*

And every now and then when I am with you
I know why I believe in angels.
When I looked in your eyes for the first time
I knew you were special.
When I rocked you at night when your pain was too much
I marveled at your courage.
And when I held you close with tears in my eyes
I knew why I believed in angels.
Charity–the pure love of Christ.
Charity–a loving sacrifice.
Unconditional love, a mission divine,
A spirit of healing from your heart to mine.
Dear Charity, I know why I believe in angels.
Before you were born you were chosen
Because of your courage.
A daughter of the morning you stood by your Lord
Witnessing of His plan.
An elect spirit, you were sent as you were
To teach us that there are angels.
Charity–the pure love of Christ
Charity–a loving sacrifice
Unconditional love, a mission divine
A spirit of healing from your heart to mine.
Dear Charity, I know why I believe in angels.
There's nothing like your smile
You gave, though it was hard
There's nothing like the love
You shared from your heart.
And though you had to go–I promise you
I'll always believe in angels.
Charity! Oh, yes, I believe in angels.

I was absolutely delighted when my friend Fred, the dishwasher from Primary Children's Medical Center, appeared at both Charity's viewing and her funeral the following day. In nearly seven years he had not changed even a little, and seemed especially pleased when my family returned his tender hugs. For a few moments he gazed at Charity's body, saying nothing. Then he began moving from one group of guests to another, hugging many and loving them all.

As so many have said about Charity, Fred too has a remarkable ability to love others. As I watched him during those two days, and as I remembered and pondered the life of my sweet daughter, I was reminded of the words of the Apostle John as recorded in the Holy Scriptures, "Beloved, let us love one another: for love is of God; and every one that loveth is born of God, and knoweth God" (1 John 4:7).

Surely, I thought as I stood by my daughter's casket and watched our young friend reaching out to others, Fred knew God. And just as surely, no one other than Christ could have exemplified and made manifest the love of God better than Fred was doing—or better than Charity had done. Seeing the results of the limitations that had kept the two of them much as little children, it is no wonder to me that God has commanded each of us to become as a little child.

Almost immediately following Charity's death we began receiving the sweetest notes and cards, many reflecting on how Charity had affected the lives of those who were writing. Despite these sweet expressions and experiences, however, once the funeral was over our home seemed to grow more empty with each passing day. Finally, unable to bear the loneliness any longer, Kathy and I threw some clothing in the car and started driving. We had no destination in mind, so we just went, talking, weeping, remembering. Never in our thirty-two years of marriage had we made such a journey, never had we spoken to each other so continuously and so openly, not just about Charity but about everything we had struggled through or enjoyed together.

For days we walked the beaches of Oregon, picking up shells, writing thank-you notes, and remembering. On the shores of Puget Sound, we watched the ferries come and go, and remembered. High in the alpine valleys of Glacier National Park, we took photographs of mountain goat nannies and their kids, wept that the sweetest little kid on earth had been called away from us, and the memories continued. Looking at the low, dry-grass hills of the Custer Battlefield on the Little Bighorn River in Montana, we thought of all the needless suffering and untimely deaths those hills had witnessed—and pondered again the one untimely death that had so devastated us. Standing beneath the looming bulks of Wyoming's Devil's Tower and South Dakota's Mount Rushmore, we considered the great works of both man and God, and again our hearts were turned to the beloved little work we had so briefly shared with heaven.

And day after day we prayed, together and alone, pleading not so much for understanding as for comfort. We both knew where our little darling had gone and were more than happy for her. What we didn't know was how to deal with the emptiness her leaving had created in our own lives.

Early one morning, perhaps two months after Charity's death, I found myself unable to sleep. Arising, I left the bedroom and slipped into an easy chair, though I was anything but relaxed. As usual I was thinking of Charity, wondering where she was, what she was doing, and if she thought as often of Kathy and me as we did of her. In short, I was wondering if she missed us or even remembered us.

Suddenly the room seemed to come alive, almost like her room had felt just before her passing. I wondered at this feeling, and then—

though I don't know if I heard this with my ears or within my mind—a sweet, feminine voice pierced the stillness, and as clearly as I have ever heard anything in my life, I heard my angel daughter say in the most loving way imaginable: *"Hi, Daddy."*

Those were the two most beautiful words I had ever heard! I wept for days afterward just thinking of their implications; I weep even now. And from that moment, I began to heal.

For Kathy, however, it was not so simple. Children and grandchildren came regularly to visit, keeping her busy and bringing much joy and happiness into our home, but as soon as they were gone, the tears of loneliness and grief resumed. She longed to see Charity, to speak with her, to have her help in sorting things out in her mind.

Then, on October 26, four months to the day from our daughter's passing, Kathy was sitting in Charity's room weeping and praying, vainly trying to find some comfort. Suddenly her mind filled with the thought that she needed to write Charity a letter. Though it was difficult, she did it, pouring out her loneliness and sorrow to her departed daughter as only a grieving mother could.

In part she wrote: "I am sitting in a room that is the nearest place to heaven I can enter. Charity, it is your sweet little room. With your favorite CD playing in the background, I feel your spirit here so strongly. Yet as I glance toward your bed there is great emptiness in my heart and soul, for you are not in it sharing your love and smiles with me anymore. . . .

"I am trying so hard, Charity, to be happy. But the tears won't go! The pain never goes away, nor the loneliness! The days since you left have been the loneliest I have ever known. Charity, I tried so hard to take perfect care of your sweet little body. You are so cute, and I always tried to keep you clean and dressed up—hair combed, teeth brushed, always looking your best. Nothing was too good for you, sweetheart. You deserved the best and more. . . .

"Oh, how I wish the tears would stop. It's no wonder, though. Heaven has been taken from us, for you were heaven, Charity. How we enjoyed that heavenly realm while you so elegantly graced our home—you and all the other beautiful angels who attended you while you were here with us.

"Charity, without ever uttering a single word you have touched the lives of thousands of people. The beautiful tributes to you at the viewing and again at the funeral were evidence of that. Your life and mission and message have all been fulfilled. How you reached out to everyone who came near you, and showed them that perfect love is somehow made most evident through imperfect—yes, and especially tattered—people.

"We can never thank you enough for coming to our home and giving us the most glorious experiences we have ever known. How I love you, my little sweetheart. I will never forget you. You'll always be our little Chare-bear. I love you forever!! Thank you for loving me and teaching me."

As she ended her poignant letter, Kathy realized that she was feeling very strongly the presence of our angelic daughter. And abruptly her mind and heart were filled with the certain knowledge that she had never been left alone at all. We were Charity's family, and our home was her home. Her love for us was as eternal as ours would be for her, and her spirit had been, and would always be, nearby.

Such understanding comforted my sweetheart immediately, and from that day she also began to heal.

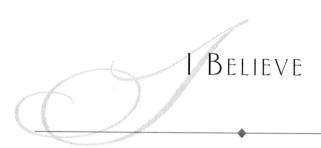

I BELIEVE

Today is Easter Sunday: March 30, 1997. There is a slight breeze this morning, but with the exception of a few thin, wispy clouds the sky is clear and brilliant blue.

I've thought constantly since little Charity Afton's passing about our experiences together, and the more I ponder, the more overwhelmed with gratitude I feel. Like anyone else, while I loved the good times and cherish the memory of her every precious smile and giggle, I would never have chosen to endure the traumatic and painful times. Yet I now believe that it took all of it—both pleasant and difficult—to instill in my family and me the repentance, the love and compassion, and the various other changes for good that her life seems to have wrought. Through all eternity I will be thankful to God for bringing her into our lives and for allowing us to cherish her as our little angel daughter.

Glancing at the calendar on my wall, I realize that it has been nine months and four days since her death. Somehow both Kathy and I have made it this far. Like millions of others before us, we have discovered that in spite of overwhelming pain and sorrow, life does go on. The long winter is mostly behind us, and outside my window nature gives glorious evidence that the earth is beginning her rebirth. The quaking aspens are already dropping their catkins or fuzzy flowers, the spruce and firs are bulging with what I know will be deliciously green candles of new growth, and everywhere bulbs have burst through the earth and are opening their petals to another spring.

Easter Sunday—a worldwide holiday celebrating the resurrection of the Lord Jesus from the cold, dark depths of his tomb. What a glorious hope this morning offers, not alone with the renewal of the earth on which we live, but with the promised renewal of all life everywhere, including that of our precious little sweetheart.

Easter Sunday. Earlier this morning, while it was yet dark, I opened the Bible and sought out the words, the passages of the promise this Easter morning holds forth to Kathy and me. As a faint light eased across the Wasatch Mountains to the east, I read of the two Marys who, in their grief, had gone early in the morning to more properly embalm the body of their crucified Lord. To their surprise and wonder, however, they found an already opened tomb, empty save for a glorious angelic being.

"And the angel answered and said unto the women, Fear not ye: for I know that ye seek Jesus, which was crucified. He is not here: for he is risen, as he said. Come, see the place where the Lord lay. And go quickly, and tell his disciples that he is risen from the dead. . . . And as they went to tell his disciples, behold, Jesus met them, saying, All hail. And they came and held him by the feet, and worshipped him" (Matthew 28:5-7, 9).

In wonder I pondered this momentous and miraculous event—this resurrection of Christ the Lord from the dead. As my room slowly filled with the light of the dawn I searched further, wanting to understand. The two Marys had held Jesus by the feet—not the feet of a spirit but those of a physical, tangible being, resurrected or raised up from the dead by the power of God, his mortal body made immortal and eternal.

In continuing witness of this, that same day in the evening the apostles had gathered together in a private room to discuss Jesus' appearance to the two women and to other disciples who had been on their way to Emmaus.

"And as they thus spake," I read next, "Jesus himself stood in the midst of them, and saith unto them, Peace be unto you. But they were terrified and affrighted, and supposed that they had seen a spirit. And he said unto them, Why are ye troubled? and why do thoughts arise in your hearts? Behold my hands and my feet, that it is I myself: handle me, and see; for a spirit hath not flesh and bones, as ye see me have. And when he had thus spoken, he shewed them his hands and his feet" (Luke 24:36–40).

Again, lest they (or I) be confused or doubt that the resurrected Lord had taken up his physical body of flesh and bones in an immortal state, the scripture continues: "And while they yet believed not for joy, and wondered, he said unto them, Have ye here any meat? And they gave him a piece of a broiled fish, and of an honeycomb. And he took it, and did eat before them" (Luke 24:41–43). Later, Peter testified of these things before the world, again reiterating that Jesus had eaten with him and the other apostles (see Acts 10:39–41).

As the first rays of the Easter morning sun strike my window I ponder these things, considering the implications. I know my beloved Charity is alive and well in the world of spirits. I know it! I have felt her presence and heard her voice. Yet with all my heart and soul I miss her beautiful little body—the tattered body of the little girl I knew—which lies in its own dark tomb. I miss holding her, touching her, loving her. I miss singing her my silly little love songs, and watching her patiently loving smile light up my life. If I were to believe that those joyous moments were over and gone forever, then I would of all men be most miserable.

But they are not! I know that, too, for this morning the Holy Spirit bears witness to my soul that it is so. As my Lord Jesus took up his once-tattered body, thus emptying his tomb as he went forth in a healed and perfected state, so, too, has he promised to bring forth Charity's body from her lonely grave.

"Marvel not at this," the beloved apostle John declared, "for the hour is coming, in the which all that are in the graves shall hear his voice, and shall come forth" (John 5:28–29).

All that are in the graves. Surely my beloved angel Charity is among the "all" who will bring forth their bodies from the grave. Then her sweet little body will no longer be tattered and dead, but she will be healed and made immortal just as Jesus was, so that in her resurrected and perfected condition she can reach up and take my hand. I can so easily envision her smiling patiently at my singing, then bursting into heavenly laughter as she skips and runs to where she can leap joyfully into the loving, waiting arms of her mother.

Oh, the joy of this sweet contemplation overwhelms me! My tears fall freely as I ponder the goodness, mercy, and grace of my Redeemer, my Savior, the Lord Jesus Christ, who also declared to me this glorious Easter morning: "I am the resurrection, and the life: he that believeth in me, though he were dead, yet shall he live: And whosoever liveth and believeth in me shall never die. Believest thou this?" (John 11:25–26).

And with all my heart and soul I answer him, "I do! Surely, my Lord, I do!"